Effective Emergency First Aid

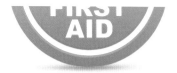

Introduction

This book has been created by experienced first aid trainers, with many years of experience, and should be used to assist you when attending a first aid training course, and in the future as a first aider.

Unfortunately, at some point in your life you may be required to deal with a real-life first aid emergency, and the question that you now need to ask yourself is:

"Will I know what to do?"

EDITION 1.1.1 **Important!**

Every casualty you may deal with will be different in numerous ways, and the medical condition, injury, or illness that they may be suffering from will differ considerably also. Therefore, the author is unable to provide a definitive guide to every situation that you may come across. As a result of this it is recommended that you seek professional medical help on all occasions, or suggest that they seek help themselves if assistance from you, the first aider, is unwanted.

After telephoning 999, or 112, for medical assistance, prompt first aid treatment of the casualty is essential to reducing the effects of any illness, or medical condition, and could save the casualty's life. Therefore, attending a recognised first aid training course, in conjunction with the use of this resource, may lead to you helping, not only yourself, but others, in your community.

Contents

The Role of the First Aider

A first-aider is someone who has undertaken training, and has a suitable qualification. This means that they must hold a valid certificate of competence in either first aid, or

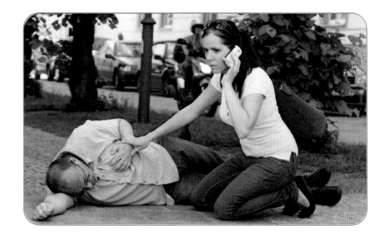

emergency first aid, issued by a reliable training organisation. An organisation should use the findings of their first-aid needs assessment to decide the level of their first aiders' knowledge, and skills, to be able to treat anyone who is injured, or becomes unwell.

To help keep the first aider's basic skills up to date, it is strongly recommended that first-aiders undertake annual refresher training.

P - Preserve Life

A first aider should preserve the casualty's life, their own, and others, until the emergency services arrive on the scene.

P - Prevent Further Injury

The first aider must take additional actions, if necessary, to prevent the incident, or situation, from becoming worse.

P - Promote Recovery

The first aider should help the casualty recover from their injury, or illness.

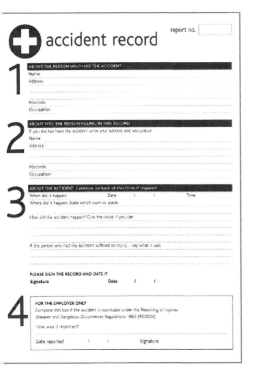

Accident Book

The accident book is a valuable document that organisations can use to record accident information as part of their management of health and safety. The following should be recorded in the accident book:

→ Details of the casualty.

→ Details of the first aider.

→ Date / time / location of the accident.

→ How the accident happened.

→ Details of the injury.

RIDDOR 1995
(Reporting of Injuries, Diseases and Dangerous Occurrences Regulations)

If you are an employer, or are in control of premises, you must report the following occurrences to the Health and Safety Executive (HSE).

→ **Deaths** *(report immediately)*

→ **Major injuries** *(report immediately)*

→ **Dangerous Occurrences** *(report immediately)*

→ **Incidents resulting in a person being off work (or unable to do full duties) for more than 7 *days*** *(report within 15 days)*

→ **Diseases** *(report as soon as possible)*

First Aid Boxes

An employer, or organisation, should provide equipment and facilities as are adequate, and appropriate, for enabling first aid to be rendered.

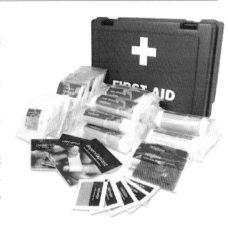

As work environments, and first aid protocols, have changed, and new first aid products have been developed, a new standard of workplace first aid kit, to help provide more effective first aid, is now available.

It is the responsibility of the first aider to replenish the first aid box immediately after every incident. First aid boxes should be located in convenient places throughout the workplace.

BS-8599 British Standard Workplace First Aid Kits

Recommended size of kit x employees	Small	Medium	Large	Vehicle
Lower Risk: e.g. Offices, shops and libraries etc.	< 25 employees	25 – 100 employees	100+ employees	Per vehicle
Higher Risk: e.g. Food processing, assembly work, Per vehicle warehousing, engineering, construction, manufacturing etc.	Less than 5 employees	5 – 25 employees	More than 25 employees	

Contents:	Small	Medium	Large	Vehicle
First aid guidance leaflet	1	1	1	1
Contents list	1	1	1	1
Nitrile disposable gloves *(pair)*	6	9	12	1
Resuscitation face shield *(with one way valve)*	1	1	2	1
Water resistant plasters *(provide blue plasters for food handlers*	40	60	100	10
Medium sterile dressings *(12cm x 12cm)*	4	6	8	1
Large sterile dressings *(18cm x 18cm)*	1	2	2	1
Eye pad sterile dressing	2	3	4	1
Finger sterile dressing	2	3	4	0
Burns dressing *(10cm x 10cm)*	1	2	2	1
Triangle bandage	2	3	4	1
Conforming bandage *(7.5cm)*	1	2	2	1
Alcohol free moist cleansing wipes	20	30	40	4
Safety pins	6	12	24	2
Adhesive tape *(2.5cm wide)*	1	1	1	1
Foil blankets	1	2	3	1
Sterile eye wash *(250ml)*	0	0	0	1
Scissors *(suitable for cutting clothes inc. leather)*	1	1	1	1

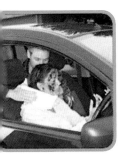

Action Plan

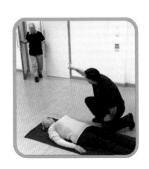

Check for dangers.
↓
Make the area safe.
↓
Shout for help.
↓
Check casualties for life threatening conditions.
↓
999 / 112.
↓
Treat casualties appropriately.
↓
Advise emergency services on their arrival.
↓
Deal with the aftermath.

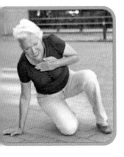

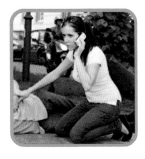

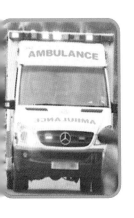

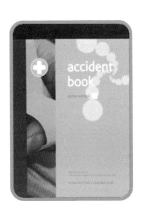

Prioritising Casualties - The Primary Survey

DR ABC

Check for **Dangers**

Check for **Response**

Check the **Airway**

Check the **Breathing**

Check for **Circulation**

Use the casualty's own body position to help promote recovery.

✓ **Shock** – Raise the casualty's legs to encourage the blood to flow to the main organs of the body, including the brain.

✓ **Faint** – Raise the casualty's legs to encourage the blood to flow to the brain.

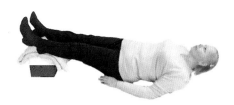

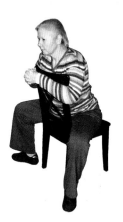

✓ **Head Injuries** – Lay the casualty down with head and shoulders raised up. Be aware that casualties with head injuries may also have neck injuries.

✓ **Stroke** – Lay the casualty down with their head and shoulders raised up.

✓ **Heart Attack** – Sit the casualty down and make them as comfortable as possible. A half sitting position is often found to be the most comfortable.

✓ **Angina** – Allow the casualty to rest in a comfortable position sitting on the floor.

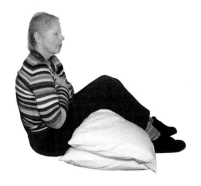

✓ **Asthma** – Help the casualty to sit upright leaning forward slightly on to the back of a chair, to allow ease of breathing.

✓ **Nose bleed** – Allow the casualty to lean forward to help prevent blood flowing down the airway.

Dealing with an Unconscious Casualty

The Recovery Position

An unconscious casualty, who is lying on their back, may have their airway blocked by either their tongue, or by vomit. To prevent the casualty's airway becoming blocked place the casualty in the "Recovery Position" as soon as possible. The vomit will then drain away out of the mouth, and the tongue will be unable to fall backwards when in the Recovery Position. Before placing the casualty in the Recovery Position, check to see if the casualty has any broken bones, or a spinal injury. The Recovery Position should be used for all casualties who have difficulty breathing, or have noisy breathing.

Step 1

→ Carefully remove the casualty's glasses, and straighten the legs out.

→ The arm nearest to you should be placed in the: "Policeman's Stop Sign."

Step 2

→ Bring the casualty's furthest away arm across their chest, holding the back of the casualty's hand against their cheek.

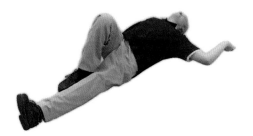

Step 3

→ With your other hand grasp the casualty's far leg, at the knee, and lift it up. The casualty's foot should remain on the floor.

→ Pull on the casualty's leg, rolling them towards you, lying them on to their side. Keep the casualty's hand pressed against their cheek.

Step 4

→ Adjust the casualty's upper leg so that both the knee, and hip, are bent at right angles. Open the casualty's airway by tilting their head back.

→ Check the casualty's breathing regularly, and commence CPR immediately, if in any doubt.

→ Call 999 / 112 for emergency help.

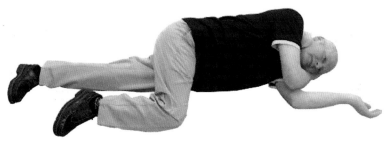

8

econdary Survey

ɘr completing a primary survey of the casualty to identify any life threatening conditions, the first aider
ɔuld call 999/112 and seek help from the emergency services. While waiting for an ambulance to arrive
 first aider should undertake a **Head to Toe Check** of the casualty, which might take about 10 minutes
ɔomplete. The purpose of this check is to try and identify further information that will be helpful to the
 ɘrgency services. Once the check has been completed, and if the ambulance has not arrived yet, then
 rt a new check of the casualty. Consider this check as a "snapshot photograph" of the casualty.

History   Is there anyone with the casualty? Have they been ill recently? Any medication ?
               Have they been to the doctors, or hospital recently?   What has happened?

Signs   What can you see? Any deformities? Any breathing difficulties? Are they alert?
               Any smell of alcohol? Are there any clues to identify the medical condition?

Symptoms   What are they telling you? Are they in any pain? How is the casualty feeling?
               "I have pains in the chest" "I feel sick" "My leg hurts" " I can't breathe properly"

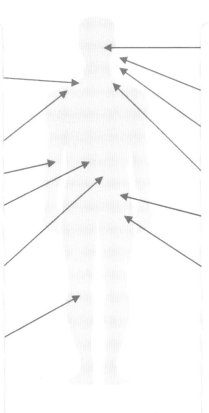

Protect the casualty's
dignity.

Talk to the casualty at all
ɼnes, and tell them who you
 re, and what you are doing.

◖Wear disposable gloves at
 ɑll times – protect yourself.

Compare shoulders and
collar bones.

ɔheck each arm individually.
Do they look similar?
Feel ribs for fractures.

Is there any bleeding?

ɼsk the casualty to breath in
ɑnd out deeply – any pain?

Broken bones?
ɔheck each leg individually.
ɔan the casualty move their
limbs – any pain?

Loosen all tight clothing.
When was their last meal?

Assess breathing.
Check pulse.

Check ears, eyes, nose,
mouth, skin, scalp, breath,
hot/cold, pale/flushed.
Compare pupil sizes.

Check the whole head.

Any swelling or bruising?
Check the neck area.

Gently feel the abdomen.
Any patterned bruising?
Any bleeding?
Incontinence?

DO NOT squeeze or rock
the pelvis.

Check for clues.
Any medic alert bracelet?
Medication.

Needle marks?
Are there any witnesses?
Be aware of "sharps."

Loss of Blood

You only have a limited amount of blood in your body, and a "Rule of Thumb" guide is **1 pint of blood** for **every stone in weight,** however, this rule does not apply if the casualty is overweight. Children, and babies, therefore, will have significantly less blood in their body to lose.

When you lose 30% of the total amount of blood in your body, serious changes may occur:
1. Blood vessels will constrict.
2. Heart rate will increase, possibly to over 100 b.p.m., and may be hard to detect.
3. Blood pressure will drop.
4. Breathing will become rapid.
5. Casualty will become restless, anxious, and may become unconscious.
6. Skin will become cold and clammy. Skin and lips will have a blue tinge (cyanosis).

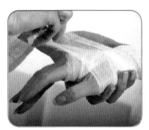 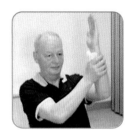 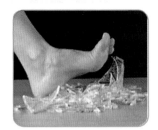

Types of wounds

Incision
This may be caused by a kitchen knife, and is usually a clean cut. This wound could bleed profusely. Blood vessels, or tendons, could be severed.

Laceration
This is a tear, or rip, of the skin. There is more likelihood that there will be dirt in the wound. Clean the wound with running water and treat for bleeding.

Abrasion
This is a graze. Likelihood of dirt in the wound. May be caused by a friction burn scraping top layers of the casualty's skin off. Clean wound thoroughly.

Contusion
Capillaries have been ruptured causing a bruise. A fracture may also have occurred. Treat by cooling the area with an ice pack.

Puncture
This may be a deep wound caused by standing on a sharp object, or maybe a stab wound. Underlying damage may have been caused. Call 999/112.

Amputation
This could be a complete, or partial, severing of a finger, toe of major limb. Call 999/112 asap. Wrap amputated part in cling film, and ice, to preserve it.

Gun Shot
Could have a small entry wound, and larger exit wound. Internal damage to organs could have been caused. Prevent blood loss. 999/112 immediately.

De-gloved
The skin has been severed from the casualty's body, exposing tissue. Replace the skin if possible. 999/112 immediately.

Shock

here are several types of Shock:

> **Hypovolaemic Shock**, when blood, or other body fluids, are lost.

> **Anaphylactic Shock,** when the heart becomes weak, blood vessels dilate, and fluid is lost.

> **Cardiogenic Shock,** when the heart does not pump the blood properly.

Signs and Symptoms

The pulse rate will increase.
Pale clammy skin - (*Check the colour of the skin inside the mouth for darker skinned casualties.*

eading on to:

Shallow, fast breathing that will rapidly get worse.
Dizziness, nausea or vomiting, weakness and sweating.
Cyanosis - (blue / grey tinge to lips and skin).

ecoming worse as the brain suffers from a reduced supply of oxygen:

Confused, becoming anxious, and on occasions becoming aggressive.
Deep, sighing breaths, as the casualty seeks out air/oxygen.
Ultimately becoming unconscious.

Treatment

Treat the cause of Shock (e,g, stop any bleeding).
Lay the casualty on the floor, and raise the casualty's legs to encourage the blood to return to the vital organs.
Keep the casualty warm, but do not overheat the casualty.
Loosen all tight clothing.
The casualty must not eat, drink or smoke.
Monitor the casualty continually, and be prepared to resuscitate the casualty if required.

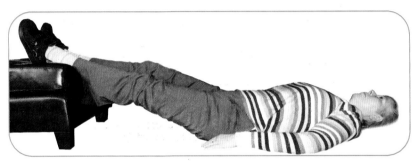

Choking – Adults and Children (1 year +)

Encourage the casualty to cough

If the choking is only mild, the casualty coughing may clear the obstruction.

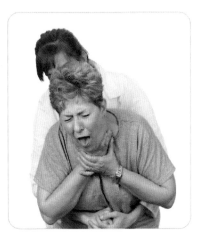

Back Blows
(Conscious casualty)

Shout for help immediately
Lean the casualty forward.

Give up to **5** back slaps between the shoulder blades.

Stop the back blows
if the obstruction clears.

Abdominal Thrusts
(Conscious casualty)

Stand behind the casualty.
Place both of your arms around the casualty's waist.

Grip your hands together below the casualty's diaphragm.

Pull inwards & upwards up to **5** times.

Stop the abdominal thrusts if the obstruction clears.

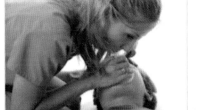

Commence C.P.R.
(Unconscious casualty)

The casualty has stopped breathing.

Call 999 / 112.

Commence CPR (30:2) and continue.

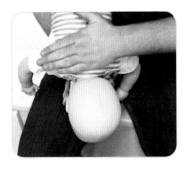

Coughing / Crying
(Conscious Casualty)

If the choking is only mild, the casualty coughing may clear the obstruction.

Back Blows
(Conscious casualty)

Shout for help immediately
Sit down / lay baby over arms.

Give up to 5 back slaps between the shoulder blades.

Stop the back blows
if the obstruction clears.

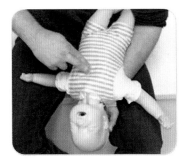

Chest Thrusts
(Conscious casualty)

Turn baby over – chest uppermost.
Using two fingers, give chest thrusts,
up to 5 times.
These thrusts are very similar to chest compressions used in CPR, but slower, and sharper. Stop chest thrusts if the obstruction clears.

Do not perform
abdominal thrusts on a baby.

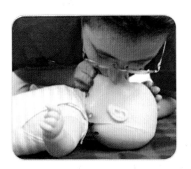

Commence C.P.R.
(Unconscious casualty)

The casualty has stopped breathing.

Call 999 / 112

Commence CPR (30:2) and continue.

Resuscitation – Sudden Collapse

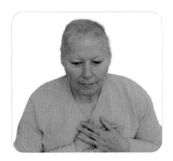

D Danger

⇩ Ensure that there are no dangers to you, the casualty, and any bystanders.

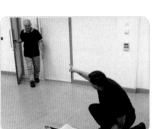

R Response

⇩ Gently shake the casualty's shoulders, and ask: "Are you alright".

If there is no response shout for help.

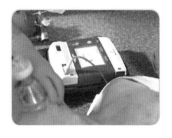

A Airway

⇩ Use **"head tilt"** and **"chin lift"** to carefully open the airway.
Place your fingers under the casualty's chin and lift.
Place your other hand on the casualty's forehead, and carefully tilt the head back.

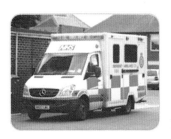

B Breathing

Check the casualty's breathing, for no more than 10 seconds.
If no breathing call for an ambulance or go yourself, if alone.
Tel: 999 / 112.
Commence with 30 compressions then 2 breaths, and repeat continually until medical help arrives.

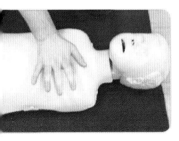

D   Danger

Ensure that there are no dangers to you, the casualty, and any bystanders

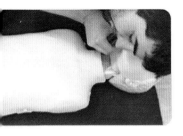

R   Response

Gently shake the casualty's shoulders, and ask "Are you alright"
If there is no response shout for help

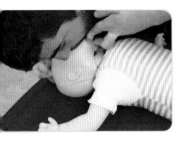

A   Airway

Use **"head tilt"** and **"chin lift"** to carefully open the airway.

Place your fingers under the casualty's chin and lift.

Place your other hand on the casualty's forehead, and carefully tilt the head back.

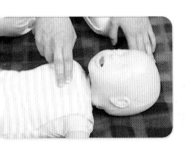

B   Breathing

Check the casualty's breathing, for no more than 10 seconds.

If no breathing call (999 / 112) or go yourself (after 1 minute's CPR if alone).

Commence with 5 initial breaths then 30 compressions and 2 breaths.

Repeat 30:2 continually until medical help arrives.

Resuscitation Techniques

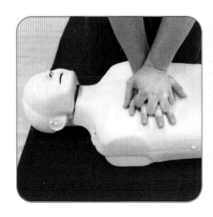

Compressions

Adults Use **2 hands** and compress 5-6 cms.
Location - centre of the chest.

Child Use **1 hand** and compress $1/3^{rd}$ of the depth of the casualty's chest.
Location - centre of the chest.

Baby Use **2 fingers** and compress $1/3^{rd}$ of the depth Of the casualty's chest.
Location – an imaginary line between the baby's nipples

"Hands Only" Cardio Pulmonary Resuscitation (CPR)

If you have not undertaken first aid training, or are unwilling, to give rescue breaths then give continuous chest compressions only.

If the casualty has suffered a "heart attack" there may be some oxygen remaining in the blood stream, and compressions will circulate that oxygen.

Continuous chest compressions should be given at the rate of 100 – 120 compressions per minute.

Do not stop resuscitation until the casualty starts breathing by themselves. If assistance is available change over every 2 minutes to prevent tiredness.

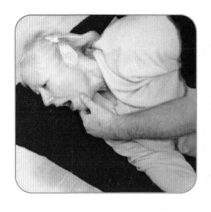

Vomiting

It is common for a casualty to vomit if they have stopped breathing after collapsing.

If the casualty vomits, quickly turn them onto their side to allow the vomit to drain out of their mouth.

Use a barrier device, or face shield, if undertaking CPR.

If there is a risk of vomiting by an unconscious casualty place the casualty in the Recovery Position.

Resuscitation Techniques

Chest does not rise

If rescue breathing does not cause the chest to rise, then reassess the degree of head tilt and chin lift being used in the resuscitation process.

No more than 2 rescue breaths should be attempted each time before returning to chest compressions. If the difficulty in rescue breathing continues, check the casualty's mouth for any visible obstruction, and remove.

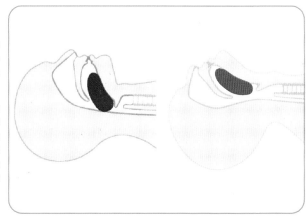

Agonal Breaths

Agonal breathing is also known as gasping for breath. It is a sign that the body is not receiving the oxygen it needs. It most often occurs when a person is actively dying. They are indicative of cardiac arrest, or the process of dying from lung cancer or emphysema.

Agonal breathing sounds like snorting, gurgling or gasping. The duration differs for each person, lasting from a few minutes, to several hours. Normal respirations are regular in regards to timing.

Agonal breathing is irregular and sporadic. It is important to remember that agonal breathing is not sufficient in delivering oxygen to the body. It is a sign of distress and is therefore not considered breathing.

Air in the stomach

If the casualty's airway is not managed correctly additional pressure during rescue breathing will be required. This may cause air to enter the stomach, and therefore unlikely that sufficient air has entered the lungs.

If swelling of the stomach occurs during resuscitation, reassess head tilt and chin lift. If a clear airway is managed, the air in the stomach will escape naturally.
DO NOT APPLY ANY PRESSURE TO THE STOMACH AREA.

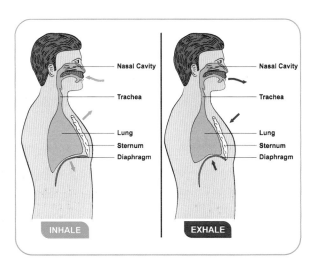

17

Dealing with Wounds

Dressings

Before applying any dressing, you should wash and dry your hands. Make sure that the casualty is sitting, or lying down. If the affected area is bleeding, it should stop if you apply pressure and raise the area higher than the heart. Use a dressing that is slightly bigger than the wound you want it to cover.

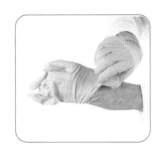

Hold the dressing at the edges, keeping your fingers away from the part that's going to cover the wound. Place the dressing on top on the wound. A little bit of pressure on the affected area should stop it from bleeding again - but make sure that you don't restrict the circulation. Sterile dressing pads come in a protective wrapping. Once they are out of the wrapping, they are no longer sterile.

When applying a sterile dressing:

✓ Hold the bandage on either side of the pad.
✓ Lay the pad directly on the wound.
✓ Wind the short end once around the limb and the pad.
✓ Wind the other end around the limb to cover the whole pad, tie the ends together over the pad to secure it, and put slight pressure on the wound.

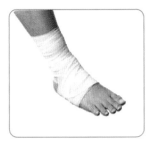

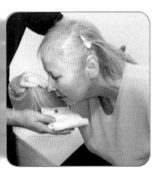

Nosebleeds

Anyone can get a nosebleed, but they most commonly occur in the following groups:
→ Young children.
→ The elderly.
→ Pregnant women.
→ People who regularly take aspirin and blood thinning medication, such as warfarin.
→ People with blood disorders.

Treating nosebleeds

✓ Sit the casualty down, with their head tipped forward.
✓ Nip the soft part of the nose, applying pressure for 10 minutes.
✓ The casualty should breathe through their mouth.
✓ Clean up blood while the nose is being nipped.
✓ Every 10 minutes release the pressure to see if the bleed has stopped.
✓ If bleeding has not stopped after a total of 20 minutes call 999/112 for an ambulance.
✓ After the bleeding has stopped advise the casualty to breathe through their nose, and not to pick or blow it, for the next 24 hours.

Dealing with Wounds

Embedded objects in the wound

Where possible, swab or wash small objects out of the wound with clean water. If there is a large object embedded:

Treatment

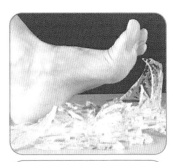

- ✓ Leave it in place.
- ✓ Apply firm pressure on either side of the object.
- ✓ Raise and support the wounded limb, or part.
- ✓ Lay the casualty down to treat for shock.
- ✓ Gently cover the wound and object with a sterile dressing.
- ✓ Build up padding around the object until the padding is higher than the object, then bandage over the object without pressing on it.
- ✓ Depending on the severity of the bleeding, dial 999 / 112 for an ambulance.
- ✓ If the casualty has got something stuck in their ear, nose, or other orifice, do not attempt to remove it. Take the casualty to hospital immediately, or call 999/112.

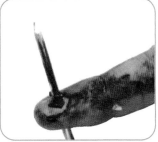

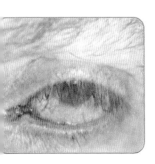

Eye Injuries

A speck of dust, a loose eyelash, or even a contact lens can float on the white of the eye. Usually, such objects can easily be rinsed off.

There may be:

→ Blurred vision.

→ Pain or discomfort.

→ Redness and watering of the eye.

→ Eyelids screwed up in spasm.

Treatment

- ✓ For a serious eye injury cover the eye with a soft sterile dressing, and bandage in place. Tell casualty to keep their injured eye closed.
- ✓ If there are chemicals, grit, or sand in the eye, wash the eye out with water, ensuring the water is poured from the bridge of the nose, and then over the injured eye. Open the casualty's eye to fully irrigate it.
- ✓ Call 999 / 112 for emergency help.

Dealing with Wounds

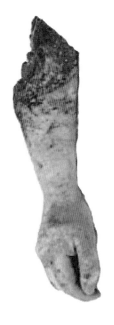

Amputation

✓ Calm and reassure the person as much as possible.
✓ Control bleeding by applying direct pressure to the wound, raise the injured area, and apply direct pressure, with help from someone who is not tired.
✓ If the person has life-threatening bleeding, a tight bandage or tourniquet will be easier to use than direct pressure on the wound. However, using a tight bandage for a long time may do more harm than good.
✓ Save any severed body parts and make sure they stay with the patient. Remove any dirty material that can contaminate the wound, if possible. Gently rinse the body part if the cut end is dirty.
✓ Wrap the severed part in a clean, damp cloth, place it in a sealed plastic bag and treat for shock.
✓ Once the bleeding is under control, check the person for other signs of injury that require emergency treatment.
✓ Do NOT directly put the body part in water without using a plastic bag.
✓ Do NOT put the severed part directly on ice.
✓ Do NOT use dry ice as this will cause frostbite and injury to the severed part.

Poisoning

A poison could be:

Corrosive
(e.g. petrol, turpentine, bleach, acids, ammonia)

Treatment:

✓ Check for dangers – is the area safe?
✓ Wash away with water if on the skin.
✓ Dilute with sips water, or milk, if swallowed. Rinse out the mouth.
✓ Identify the poison, or chemical if possible.
✓ Call 999 / 112 for emergency help as soon as possible.

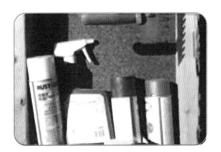

Non-Corrosive
(e.g. plants, berries, tablets, alcohol, drugs)

Treatment:

✓ Identify the poison if possible.
✓ Call 999 / 112 for emergency help as soon as possible.

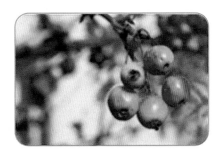

Sprains, Strains and Dislocations

Sprains

A sprain occurs when one or more of your ligaments have been stretched, twisted or torn, usually as a result of excessive force being applied to a joint.
The most common locations for a sprain to occur are:
- → **the knee**
- → **the ankle**
- → **the wrist**
- → **the thumb**

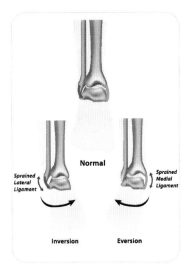

Strains

A strain occurs when the muscle fibres stretch, or tear. They usually occur when the muscle has been stretched beyond its limits, or it has been forced to contract (shorten) too quickly.
Strains can develop as the result of an accident, or during physical activities, such as running or playing football.
The most common types of strains are:
- → Hamstring.
- → Calf.
- → Thigh.
- → Lower back.

Treatment

- ✓ **Rest** - rest the injured area.
- ✓ **Ice** - apply an ice pack to the injured area.
- ✓ **Comfortable Support** - apply a firm dressing to reduce swelling.
- ✓ **Elevation** - elevate the injury.

Normal

Sprained Lateral Ligament

Sprained Medial Ligament

Inversion

Eversion

Dislocations

Dislocations are joint injuries that force the ends of your bones out of position. The cause is often a fall or a blow, sometimes from playing a contact sport. When a dislocation occurs, you can't move the joint. You can dislocate your ankles, knees, shoulders, hips and elbows. You can also dislocate your finger and toe joints. Dislocated joints often are swollen, very painful and visibly out of place.
When properly repositioned, a joint will usually function and move normally again in a few weeks.

Treatment

- ✓ Immobilise.
- ✓ Call 999 / 112 for emergency services.

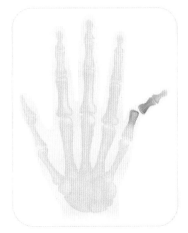

Burns and Scalds

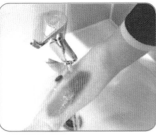

Appropriate first aid must be used to treat any burns or scalds as soon as possible. This will limit the amount of damage caused to the skin.

Treatment

Stop the burning process as soon as possible. This may mean removing the person from the area, dousing flames with water, or smothering flames with a blanket. Do not put yourself at risk of getting burnt as well.

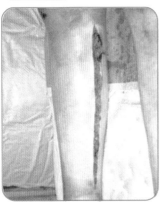

Remove any clothing, or jewellery, near the burnt area of skin. However, don't try to remove anything that is stuck to the burnt skin because this could cause more damage.

Cool the burn with cool or lukewarm water for 10–30 minutes, at least, ideally within 20 minutes of the injury occurring. Never use ice, iced water or any creams or greasy substances, such as butter.

Keep the casualty warm. Use a blanket, or layers of clothing, but avoid putting them on the injured area. Keeping warm will prevent hypothermia. This is a risk if you are cooling a large burnt area, particularly in young children and elderly people.

Cover the burn with cling film. Put the cling film in a layer over the burn, rather than wrapping it around a limb. A clean, clear plastic bag can be used for burns on your hand.

✓ **Get medical help straight away if the person with the burn:**

- Has other injuries that need treating, or is going into shock.
- Is pregnant.
- Is over 60 years of age.
- Is under five years of age.
- Has a medical condition such as heart, lung or liver disease, or diabetes.
- Has a weakened immune system.

✓ **Call 999 / 112 for:**

- All chemical and electrical burns.
- Large or deep burns – any burn bigger than the affected person's hand.
- Full thickness burns of all sizes – these burns cause white or charred skin.
- Partial thickness burns on the face, hands, arms, feet, legs or genitals – these are burns that cause blisters.

Superficial burn 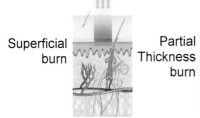 Partial Thickness burn 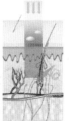 Full Thickness burn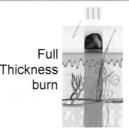

Anaphylaxis

Introduction

A severe allergic reaction will affect the whole body, in susceptible individuals it may develop within seconds of contact with the trigger factor, and is potentially fatal.

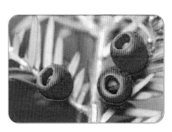

Possible triggers can include skin or airborne contact with particular materials, the injection of a specific drug, the sting of a certain insect or the ingestion of a food such as peanuts.

Recognition features

→ Impaired breathing: this may range from a tight chest to severe difficulty in breathing.
→ There may be a wheeze or gasping for air.
→ Signs of shock.
→ Widespread blotchy skin eruption.
→ Swelling of the tongue and throat.
→ Puffiness around the eyes.
→ Anxiety.

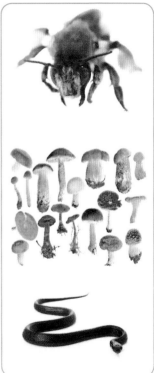

Treatment

Your aim is to arrange immediate removal of the casualty to hospital. Dial 999 or 112 for the emergency services.

✓ Give any information you have on the cause of the casualty's condition.

✓ Check whether the casualty is carrying any necessary medication. If they are, help them to use it.

✓ If the casualty is conscious help them to sit up in a position that most relieves any breathing difficulty; this is usually sitting up and leaning forward slightly.

If the casualty becomes unconscious:

✓ Open the airway and check breathing.

✓ Be prepared to give rescue breaths and chest compressions.

✓ Place them into the recovery position if the casualty is unconscious but breathing normally.

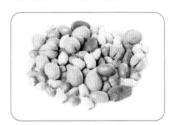

Broken Bones

The Skeleton

→ Consisting of 206 bones.

→ Protects vital organs.

→ Stores calcium, fats and minerals.

→ Provides support for the soft tissue.

→ Gives the body its shape.

→ Produces blood cells and platelets.

→ Allows movement using various joints, and muscle attachment.

Causes of fractures

→ Direct force
(Injury is caused at the area where force was applied)

→ Indirect force
(Injury is caused away from the area where force was applied.)

→ Pathological
(Injury is caused because of weak, and/or brittle bones).

→ Violent movement
(Injury is caused due to sudden and violent movements)

→ Twisting forces
(Injury is caused due to torsion on the bones).

Signs and symptoms

→ Loss of power.

→ Bruising and/or swelling.

→ Irregularity.

→ Tenderness.

→ Pain.

→ Unnatural movement.

→ Deformity.

→ Crepitus.

Treatment

✓ Immobilise the fracture.

✓ Calm and reassure the casualty.

✓ Keep the casualty warm.

✓ Call 999 / 112 an ambulance.

X Do not move the casualty, unless they are in danger.

X Do not bandage the casualty if the ambulance has been called for.

X Do not give the casualty anything to eat or drink.

Common types of fracture

Open	Closed	Comminuted	Greenstick

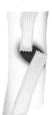
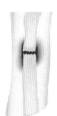
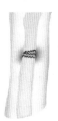
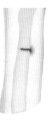

Spinal Injuries

Signs and symptoms

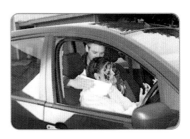

The spine, or backbone, protects the spinal cord, which controls many body functions. Back injuries can be caused by pinching or displacement of nerves, or by a spinal fracture.

Suspect a spinal injury after an awkward fall or awkward injury. These injuries could also include:

→ Diving in to shallow water.

→ Falling from a height.

→ Being involved in a car accident.

→ A blow to the head, neck, and/or back.

→ Crush injuries.

Look for:

→ Localised tenderness around the back or neck.

→ Shooting pains in the casualty's limbs.

→ Limbs feeling heavy or tingling.

→ Loss of sensation in the limbs below level of injury.

→ Breathing difficulties.

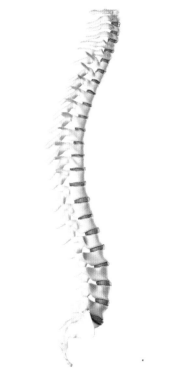

Treatment

✓ Calm the casualty, ask them not to move, and keep them warm.

✓ Do not move the casualty, unless they are in danger.

✓ Keep the casualty in the position you found them.

✓ Support the head, and try and keep it in line with the upper body.

✓ Call 999 / 112 for the emergency services.

✓ If the casualty is unconscious try and maintain an open airway.

✓ If CPR is required to be undertaken you may have to tilt the head back slightly, and lift the chin, to open the airway.

✓ If the casualty vomits, or you need to put the casualty in to the Recovery Position you must try and keep the head in line with the upper body when you turn the casualty. Get help, if available, to perform this task.

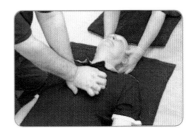

Heart Attack / Angina

Heart Attack

The heart beats on average 60 – 80 beats a minute to push blood around the body. Like any busy muscle, the heart tissues need a good supply of blood from their blood vessels, which are called the coronary arteries. When this process is interrupted or doesn't work properly, serious illness and even death can result.

A heart attack occurs when blood flow to part of the heart is blocked, often by a blood clot, causing damage to the affected muscle.

If blood supply is cut off for a long time, the muscle cells are irreversibly damaged and die, leading to disability or death depending on the extent of the damage.

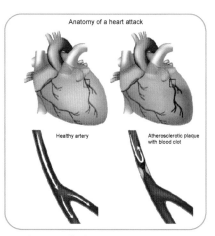

Anatomy of a heart attack

Healthy artery

Atherosclerotic plaque with blood clot

Signs & Symptoms for Heart Attack and Angina

Every heart attack is different, and not all signs and symptoms are present. The main difference between a heart attack, and angina, could be as simple as the duration of pain.

	Angina	Heart Attack
Onset	Sudden. During exercise. Stress. Arguments. Extreme weather.	Sudden. Can occur while resting. Sometimes no warning sign.
Pain	Can be mistaken for indigestion. "Vice-like squashing pain. A dull tightness, or pressure.	Can be mistaken for indigestion. "Vice-like squashing pain. A dull tightness, or pressure.
Area of pain	Centre of the chest initially, but will radiate out to the neck, shoulders, jaw, back and arms (usually left arm).	Centre of the chest initially, but will radiate out to the neck, shoulders, jaw, back and arms (usually left arm).
Skin	Pale, and the casualty may be sweating.	Grey colour / pale, and the casualty may be sweating profusely.
Pulse Rate	May become irregular, and missing beats.	May become irregular, and missing beats.
Other Signs & Symptoms	Anxiety, weakness, shortness of breath.	Dizziness, nausea, vomiting, shortness of breath, and a sense of impending doom.
Duration of pain	Pain will usually last between 3 to 8 minutes. Very rarely longer.	Pain will usually last for longer than 30 minutes.
Relief Factors	If casualty rests it will give relief. G.T.N. spray / medication.	G.T.N. spray / medication may give the casualty some relief.

Angina

Angina develops when the muscles of the heart are not getting enough oxygen; this is usually caused by narrowing or blockages of the coronary arteries that deliver oxygen-rich blood to the heart muscle, known as coronary artery disease. Angina is a sign of heart disease.

If the blockage of a coronary artery progresses and becomes complete, the blood supply to part of the muscles of the heart is lost, causing a heart attack. Angina is a warning sign. One patient in 10 will go on to have a heart attack within a year of diagnosis of angina.

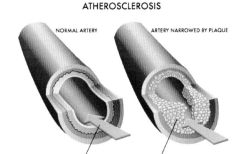

ATHEROSCLEROSIS

NORMAL ARTERY   ARTERY NARROWED BY PLAQUE

BLOOD FLOW   ATHEROSCLEROTIC PLAQUE

Treatment for Heart Attack and Angina

The treatment for both Angina and Heart Attack are very similar, however, Angina pain will usually subside within 3 – 8 minutes if the casualty rests.

✓	Sit the casualty in a comfortable position. Do not allow the casualty to move around. A half sitting position is considered to be the best. (The "W" position). Call **999 / 112** for the emergency services.
✓	Calm and reassure the casualty. Remove all causes of stress, or anxiety, for the casualty. Allow the casualty to take any medication that they have e.g. glyceryl tri-nitrate (G.T.N.) medication / spray.
✓	If you suspect a heart attack, and the casualty is over 16 years of age, and not allergic, allow them to slowly chew on an Aspirin, to assist in reducing any damage to the heart.
✓	Monitor the casualty continuously. If a heart attack casualty becomes unconscious then the heart may have stopped altogether, so you should be ready to deliver CPR.
✓	Call **999 / 112** for the emergency services if the situations worsens, or: - a heart attack is suspected. - the Angina sufferers symptoms are different, or worse, than normal. - The Angina pain is not relieved by either resting, or using their medication. - The casualty has never been diagnosed with Angina in the past. - Angina pain has commenced during sleep, or whilst at rest. - You are in any doubt about the casualty's condition
✓	N.B. A first aider is never allowed to prescribe drugs to a casualty. However, if the casualty is conscious the casualty can decide for themselves whether to take any form of medication for themselves, or not.
✓	N.B. Aspirin will reduce the clotting ability of the blood. If the casualty chews the Aspirin it will allow absorption quickly into the blood stream through the skin inside the mouth. (A 300mg dose of Aspirin is sufficient, but any dosage will do)

Diabetes

Diabetes occurs when the body can't use glucose properly, either owing to a lack of the hormone insulin or because the insulin available doesn't work effectively.

It is estimated that more than two million people in the UK have the condition and up to 750,000 more are believed to have it but without realising they do.

More than three-quarters of people with diabetes have Type 2 Diabetes. The number of people with Type 2 Diabetes is rapidly increasing as it is more common in the overweight and obese, which is itself a growing problem.

The remainder have type 1 diabetes mellitus, which used to be known as insulin-dependent diabetes mellitus.

Type 1 Diabetes
In type 1 diabetes, the body is unable to produce any insulin.
It usually starts in childhood or young adulthood, and is treated with diet control and insulin injections.

Type 2 Diabetes
In Type 2 Diabetes, not enough insulin is produced or the insulin that is made by the body doesn't work properly.
It tends to affect people as they get older and usually appears after the age of 40, but increasingly is seen in younger, overweight people.

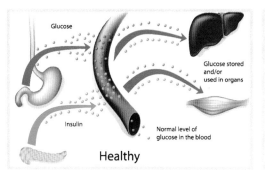

Healthy

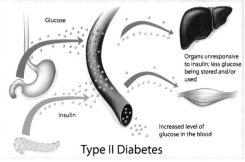

Type II Diabetes

Signs and Symptoms

→ A history of diabetes.

→ Weakness, faintness, or hunger.

→ Palpitations and muscle tremors.

→ Strange actions or behaviour; confusion or belligerence.

→ Sweating and cold, clammy skin.

→ Pulse may be rapid and strong.

→ Deteriorating level of response.

→ Diabetic's warning card, glucose gel, tablets, or an insulin syringe.

Treatment

✓ Raise the sugar content of the blood as quickly as possible.

✓ Help the casualty to sit or lie down.

✓ Give them a sugary drink, sugar lumps or sweet food.

✓ Give them more food and drink and let them rest until they feel better.

✓ Advise them to see their doctor even if they feel fully recovered.

✓ If the casualty does not respond call 999 / 112 for the emergency services.

erious Head Injuries

Fractured Skull

The most common signs and symptoms of a fractured skull are:

→ Wound or bruise on the head, soft area or depression on the scalp.

→ Bruising or swelling behind one ear, and around one or both eyes.

→ Clear fluid or watery blood coming from the nose or an ear.

→ Blood in the white of the eye.

→ Distortion or lack of symmetry of the head or face.

→ Progressive deterioration in the level of response.

Concussion

The most common signs and symptoms of concussion are:

→ Headache, dizziness, nausea.

→ Confusion, such as being unaware of your surroundings

→ Feeling stunned or dazed.

→ Disturbances with vision, double vision or flashing lights.

→ Difficulties with memory.

→ Loss of balance.

Compression

The most common signs and symptoms of compression are:

→ History of a recent head injury, and an intense headache.

→ Noisy breathing, becoming slow, and drowsiness.

→ Slow, yet full and strong pulse and an unequal pupil size.

→ Weakness and/or paralysis down one side of the face of body.

→ High temperature and a flushed face.

→ Noticeable change in personality or behaviour, such as irritability.

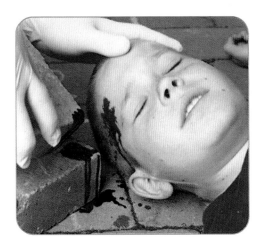

Treatment for head injuries

If the casualty is conscious:

✓ Help them to lie down. **Do not** turn the head in case there is a neck injury.

✓ Control any bleeding from the scalp by applying pressure around the wound.

✓ Look for and treat any other injuries. **Dial 999 / 112** for the emergency services.

✓ If there is discharge from an ear, cover the ear with a sterile dressing or clean pad, lightly secured with a bandage. **Do not plug the ear.**

✓ Monitor and record vital signs – level of response, pulse, and breathing.

If the casualty is unconscious:

✓ Open the airway and check for breathing (primary survey).

✓ Be prepared to give chest compressions and rescue breaths if needed.

✓ **Dial 999** for the emergency services.

✓ If the position in which the casualty was found prevents maintenance of an open airway or you fail to open it, place the casualty in the recovery position. If you have helpers, use the 'log-roll" technique.

Stroke

A stroke is a serious medical condition that occurs when the blood supply to part of the brain is cut off.
Strokes are a medical emergency, and prompt treatment is essential because the sooner a person receives treatment for a stroke, the less damage is likely to happen.

If you suspect that someone is having a stroke, phone 999 / 112 immediately and ask for an ambulance.

Like all organs, the brain needs the oxygen and nutrients provided by blood to function properly. If the supply of blood is restricted or stopped, brain cells begin to die. This can lead to brain damage and possibly death.

There are two main causes of strokes:

→   Ischaemic (80% of all cases) – the blood supply is stopped due to a blood clot.

→   Haemorrhagic – a weakened blood vessel supplying the brain bursts and causes brain damage.

There is also a related condition known as a transient Ischaemic attack (TIA), where the supply of blood to the brain is temporarily interrupted, causing a 'mini-stroke'. TIAs should be treated seriously as they are often a warning sign that a stroke is coming.

Signs and symptoms

Act FAST if you suspect a stroke has occurred:

F   Facial Weakness

A   Arm Weakness

S   Speech Problems

T   Time to call 999 / 112

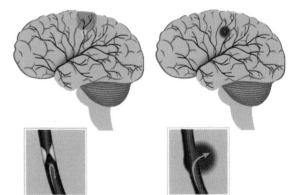

Other signs and symptoms could be:

→   Loss of balance.
→   Unequal pupil sizes.
→   Confusion.
→   Problems with sight.
→   Severe headache.
→   Numbness of the face.

Ischaemic Stroke   Haemorrhagic Stroke

Treatment for Stroke

✓   Monitor the casualty's airway, and breathing.
✓   Calm and reassure the casualty. Call 999 / 112 and ask for the emergency services.
✓   Lay a conscious casualty down and raise the their head and shoulders up.
✓   Place an unconscious casualty in to the recovery position.
✓   Monitor the casualty's breathing, pulse and their levels of response.

Seizures

A seizure – also called a convulsion, or fit – consists of involuntary contractions of many muscles in the body. The condition is due to a disturbance in the electrical activity of the brain. Seizures usually result in loss or impairment of consciousness. The most common cause is epilepsy.

Other causes include:

→ Head injury.

→ Some brain damaging diseases.

→ Shortage of oxygen or glucose in the brain.

→ The intake of certain poisons including alcohol.

Epileptic seizures are due to recurrent, major disturbances of brain activity. These seizures can be sudden and dramatic. Just before a seizure, a casualty may have a brief warning period (aura) with, for example, a strange feeling or a special smell or taste.

Signs and symptoms

→ Sudden unconsciousness; Rigidity and arching of the back; Convulsive movements.

In epilepsy the following sequence is common:

→ The casualty suddenly falls unconscious, often letting out a cry. They become rigid, arching their back.

→ Breathing may cease. The lips may show a grey-blue tinge (cyanosis) and the face and neck may become red and puffy.

→ Convulsive movements begin. The jaw may be clenched and breathing may be noisy. Saliva may appear at the mouth and may be blood-stained if the lips or tongue have been bitten. There may be loss of bladder or bowel control.

→ Muscles relax and breathing becomes normal; the casualty recovers consciousness, usually within a few minutes. They may feel dazed or act strangely. They may be unaware of their actions.

→ After a seizure, the casualty may feel tired and fall into a deep sleep.

Treatment

✓ If you see the casualty falling, try to ease the fall.

✓ Make space around them; ask bystanders to move away.

✓ Remove potentially dangerous items, such as hot drinks and sharp objects.

✓ Note the time when the seizure started.

✓ If possible, protect the casualty's head by placing soft padding underneath it.

✓ Loosen clothing around the neck.

Caution!

● Do not move the casualty unless they are in immediate danger.

● Do not put anything in their mouth or use force to restrain them.

Warning!

If any of the following apply, dial 999 for an ambulance.

● The casualty is unconscious for more than 10 minutes.

● The seizure continues for more than 5 minutes.

● The casualty is having repeated seizures or having their first seizure.

● The casualty is not aware of any reason for the seizure.

Asthma

In an asthma attack the muscles of the air passages in the lungs go into spasm and the linings of the airways swell. As a result, the airways become narrowed and breathing becomes difficult.

Sometimes there is a specific trigger for an asthma attack such as:
→ An allergy
→ A cold
→ Cigarette smoke
→ Extremes of temperature
→ Exercise.

People with asthma usually deal well with their own attacks by using a blue reliever inhaler.

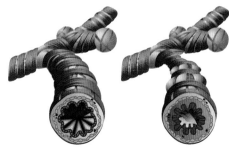

Normal bronchiole   **Asthmatic bronchiole**

Signs and Symptoms

→ Difficulty in breathing, with a very prolonged breathing-out phase.

There may also be:

→ Wheezing as the casualty breathes out.
→ Difficulty speaking and whispering.
→ Distress and anxiety.
→ Coughing.
→ Features of hypoxia, such as a grey-blue tinge to the lips, and earlobes (cyanosis).

Treatment

Your aims during an asthma attack are to ease the breathing and if necessary get medical help.

✓ You need to keep the casualty calm and reassure them.
✓ If they have a blue reliever inhaler then encourage them to use it.
✓ Encourage the casualty to breathe slowly and deeply.
✓ Encourage the casualty to sit in a position that they find most comfortable.
✓ A mild asthma attack should ease within three minutes but if it doesn't encourage the casualty to use their inhaler again.

Caution!

If this is the first attack, or if the attack is severe and any one of the following occurs:

● The inhaler has no effect after five minutes.
● The casualty is becoming worse.
● Breathlessness makes talking difficult.
● The casualty becomes exhausted.

Dial 999 / 112 for an ambulance

Warning!

● Encourage the casualty to use their inhaler every 5 - 10 minutes.
● Monitor and record the breathing and pulse rate every 10 minutes.

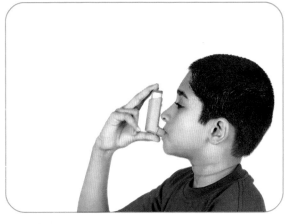

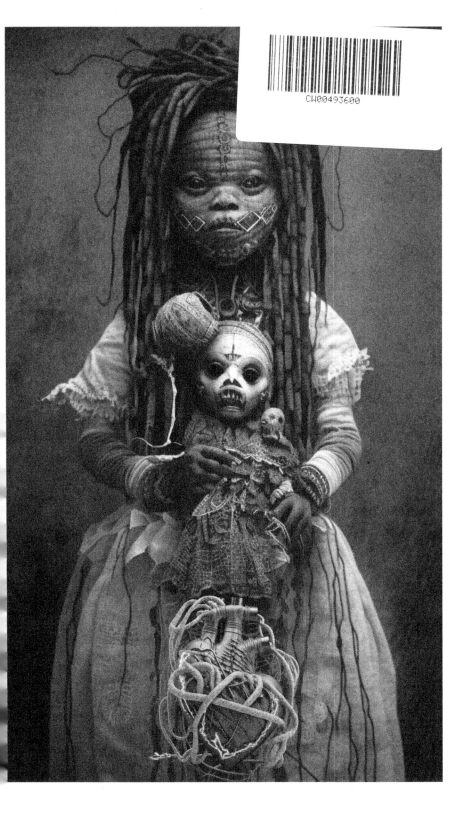

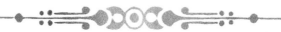

Disclaimer

The information contained in this voodoo spell book is provided for entertainment purposes only. The author and publisher of this book do not endorse or condone the use of voodoo spells for any harmful or illegal activities. The spells in this book should only be used with the utmost caution and at your own risk.

The spells contained in this book are based on traditional voodoo practices and are provided as historical and cultural information. The author and publisher of this book make no claims as to the effectiveness or safety of these spells.

The use of any spell in this book is entirely at the user's discretion. The author and publisher of this book assume no responsibility for any consequences that may result from the use of these spells.

Furthermore, this book is copyrighted material, and all rights are reserved. No part of this book may be reproduced or transmitted in any form or by any means, electronic or mechanical, including photocopying, recording, or by any information storage and retrieval system, without permission in writing from the author and publisher.

Unauthorized copying, distribution, or use of any spells in this book will result in a curse so terrible, it'll make your head spin like a voodoo doll.

By purchasing this book, you agree to never attempt to make a copy of it, unless you want to be haunted by the ghost of a lawyer for the rest of your days.

Any unauthorized use of the content in this book is strictly prohibited and may result in legal action. All rights reserved © 2023

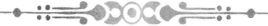

CONTENTS

CONTENTS

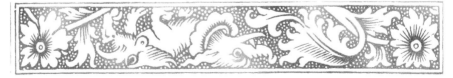

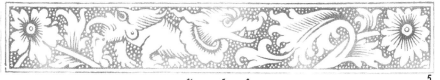

Voodoo, also known as Vodou or Vodun, is a religion and belief system that originated in West Africa and was brought to the Caribbean and the Americas during the era of the slave trade. The practice of voodoo has a rich and complex history, filled with twists and turns, triumphs and tragedies, and a deep connection to the human experience.

The roots of voodoo can be traced back to the ancient kingdoms of West Africa, where various tribal groups practiced their own forms of ancestor worship, animism, and spirit possession. As these tribes were uprooted and forcibly brought to the New World, they brought with them their religious beliefs and practices, which eventually blended together to form the syncretic religion of voodoo.

In the Caribbean, voodoo became intertwined with the practices of the slave trade, as Africans were brought to work on sugar plantations and other colonial enterprises. Slaves were forced to adopt the religion of their masters, but they also found ways to keep their own traditions alive. Voodoo became a way for slaves to maintain their cultural identity and resist the dehumanizing conditions of slavery.

Despite its enduring popularity, voodoo has also faced its fair share of persecution and misunderstanding. In the early 20th century, many voodoo practitioners were targeted by the police and the church, who saw the religion as a threat to social order.

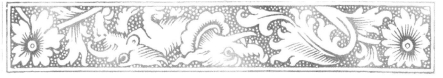

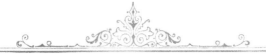

SPELLBINDING KISSES

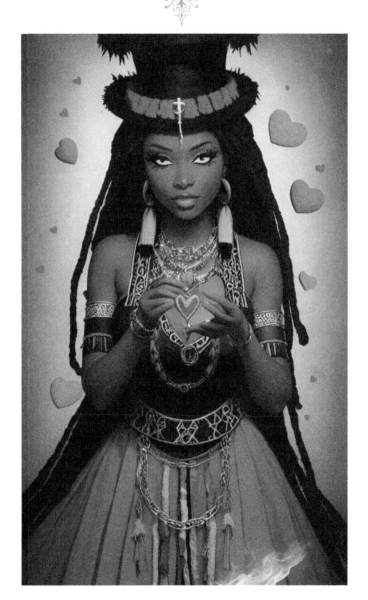

OBSESSION'S FIRE SPELL

Obsession's Fire Spell is a powerful voodoo magic spell designed to ignite intense feelings of love and desire in the target's heart. It is known for its ability to create an unbreakable bond between two people. If you want to use this spell, you must be fully aware of the consequences of your actions, as it is not reversible.

The spell is said to have originated in the deep forests of Haiti, where voodoo practitioners have been practicing their craft for centuries. According to legend, the spell was first used by a young woman named Marie, who was deeply in love with a man named Henri. However, Henri was already engaged to another woman, and Marie knew that her chances of winning him over were slim. In desperation, she turned to a voodoo priestess, who taught her the secrets of the spell.

Marie performed the spell with great care and soon noticed a change in Henri's behavior. He became more attentive to her, more loving, and more devoted. It was as if he couldn't get enough of her. But the spell had unintended consequences. Henri's fiancée soon found out about their affair and confronted him. In a fit of rage, Henri killed his fiancée and was eventually caught by the authorities and executed.

Consumed with guilt, Marie went into hiding and was never seen again.

You will need the following:

- One red candle
- A piece of paper with the target's name written on it in red ink
- A drop of your own blood
- Dragon's blood incense
- A piece of red cloth
- A red ribbon
- A lock of the target's hair
- A handful of rose petals

To perform the spell, follow these steps:

1. Light the Dragon's blood incense and let it burn while you prepare the other ingredients.
2. Light the red candle and focus your mind on the target while holding the paper with their name on it.
3. Prick your finger with a needle and let a drop of your blood fall onto the paper.
4. Chant the following incantation: "By the power of fire and blood, I call upon the spirits above, To ignite the flames of desire, In the heart of my one true love."
5. Place the lock of hair and rose petals on the paper and wrap it up in the red cloth, securing it with the ribbon.
6. Hold the package in your hands and visualize the target falling madly in love with you. Imagine the two of you together, happy and in love.
7. Place the package near the burning incense and let it burn down completely.
8. Once the fire has consumed the package, bury the ashes under a tree.

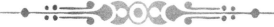

RED HEART PASSION SPELL

The Red Heart Passion Spell is a powerful voodoo love spell that can help bring new passion and excitement into an existing relationship or ignite a spark of romance between two people who have yet to discover each other. This spell uses the heart's power and the color red's intense energy to invoke feelings of love, desire, and lust.

Legend has it that the Red Heart Passion Spell was created by a powerful voodoo priestess who lived deep in the heart of the Louisiana bayou. She was known for her incredible beauty and her intense passion, and many men came to her seeking her love and affection. However, the priestess was very selective in her choice of lovers, and she would often turn away those who did not meet her high standards.

One day, a young man came to the priestess, begging for her love. His handsome features and charming personality immediately took her, and she agreed to take him on as her lover. However, the young man soon proved unfaithful, and the priestess was heartbroken.

Determined to win back her lover's affection, the priestess turned to voodoo magic. She crafted a powerful spell using the color red and the energy of the heart, and she cast the spell over the young man. To her surprise, the spell worked like a charm, and the young man was once again completely devoted to her.

Word of the priestess's incredible love spell soon spread throughout the bayou, and many people came to her seeking her help in heart matters. She taught them the Red Heart Passion Spell.

As time passed, the couple grew closer, and their love continued to burn bright. However, the man's jealousy grew stronger every day. He became possessive and controlling, preventing his lover from seeing friends and family. Eventually, the woman realized that his love had turned into an unhealthy obsession.

Desperate to break free from his grip, she sought the help of a voodoo priestess who knew of the Red Heart Passion Spell. The priestess agreed to help the woman but warned her of the consequences of using such a powerful spell. Undeterred, the woman was willing to do anything to escape her lover's grasp.

The priestess began preparing the spell's ingredients, carefully selecting the finest quality herbs and oils. The woman was instructed to light the red candles, anoint herself with the oils, and recite the incantation while focusing her energy on breaking free from her lover's hold. As she spoke the words, the flames of the candles grew brighter and hotter until they were a deep crimson.

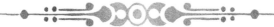

Suddenly, the woman felt a jolt of pain shoot through her heart. She stumbled backward and clutched her chest, gasping for air. As she looked up, she saw her lover's face also twisted in pain. At that moment, she realized that the spell had not only broken his hold on her but had also bound their hearts together forever.

The woman and her former lover were now inexplicably connected by an unbreakable bond of passion and desire. They could not be apart for more than a few hours without feeling an unbearable ache in their chests. The woman had unknowingly created a spell that had gone far beyond her intentions and bound them together in a way neither could have predicted.

The couple decided to make the best of their situation and dedicated their lives to studying and understanding the power of voodoo magic. They became renowned practitioners and shared their knowledge with others, always warning of the dangers of spells like the Red Heart Passion Spell.

To this day, their love burns as hot as the flames of the candles that ignited their passion all those years ago. And though they are bound together forever, they have found a way to live in harmony and use their gift to help others find love and happiness.

You will need the following:

- A red candle
- A piece of parchment paper
- A pen with red ink
- Red rose petals
- A small red bag or pouch

To perform the spell, follow these steps:

1. Begin by finding a quiet, private space where you can perform the spell undisturbed. Sit or stand in front of a table, altar, or other flat surfaces where you can place your materials.
2. Light the red candle and take a few deep breaths to ground yourself and connect with your intention. Focus your thoughts on the person you desire or the person with whom you wish to rekindle the passion.
3. Take the piece of parchment paper and write the name of the person you desire in red ink. Be sure to write their name as clearly and legibly as possible, and try to infuse each letter with your intent and desire.
4. Sprinkle the red rose petals over the parchment paper. As you do so, visualize your love and passion for this person growing and intensifying like a flame that burns brighter with every petal that falls.
5. Fold the parchment paper in half, ensuring the rose petals are tucked safely inside. Please fold the paper in half again, and continue folding until it is small enough to fit inside the red bag or pouch.
6. Hold the red bag or pouch in your hand and speak the following incantation:

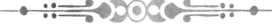

7. "Red hearts beat as one. Passion, desire, and love we've won. In this bag, I seal my intent, To bring (name of person) to me, heaven-sent."
8. Once you have spoken the incantation, place the folded parchment paper inside the bag or pouch. Hold the pouch in your hands and visualize the person you desire coming closer and closer to you until they are standing right in front of you.
9. Blow out the red candle, and carry the red bag or pouch with you wherever you go, knowing that the spell is working its magic to bring you closer to the one you desire.

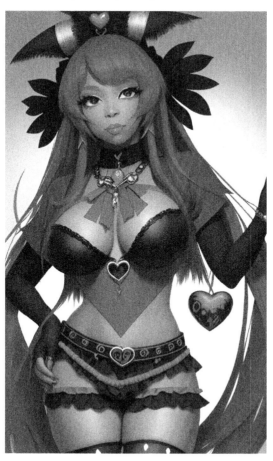

DEVOTION'S ETERNAL FLAME SPELL

Devotion's Eternal Flame Spell is a powerful voodoo spell designed to ignite an eternal flame of love and dedication in the heart of your desired one. This spell is not to be taken lightly as it requires a great deal of focus and energy to cast. The ingredients for this spell must be gathered during the full moon, which is the peak of the lunar cycle and the most potent time for spellcasting.

The Devotion's Eternal Flame Spell has a long and storied history in the practice of voodoo magic. According to legend, the spell was first cast by a powerful voodoo priestess named Marie Laveau in New Orleans in the 19th century. Marie was known for her incredible spellcasting abilities and her ability to heal the sick and mend broken hearts.

One day, a young woman came to Marie seeking help with a broken heart. She had been deeply in love with a man who had since left her for another woman. Marie listened carefully to the woman's story and decided to cast a spell to ignite an eternal flame of love and devotion in the man's heart, bringing him back to the woman forever.

Marie gathered the ingredients needed for the spell and cast it under the full moon's light. The spell worked like a charm, and the man returned to the woman, his heart burning with a new flame of devotion that could never be extinguished. From that

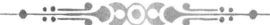

day forward, Marie's Devotion's Eternal Flame Spell became one of the most sought-after spells in the world of voodoo magic.

You will need the following:

- A red candle
- A white candle
- A piece of parchment paper
- A pen or marker
- Rose petals
- Lavender oil
- A small jar with a lid

To perform the spell, follow these steps:

1. Begin by lighting both candles and placing them in front of you. The red candle represents passion and desire, while the white candle represents purity and devotion.
2. On the piece of parchment paper, write the name of the person you desire to ignite eternal devotion in. Be sure to write their full name in clear, legible handwriting.
3. Sprinkle rose petals on top of the parchment paper and fold it in half, making sure the petals are securely inside.
4. Hold the folded paper in your hand and close your eyes. Visualize the person you desire standing in front of you, and see their heart opening up to you.
5. Anoint the red candle with lavender oil and light it. Hold the folded paper in the flame and say the following incantation: "By the light of this flame, I call upon the forces of the universe to ignite the eternal flame of love and devotion in the heart of (name of desired person). May their heart open up to me and forever burn with the flame of our love."

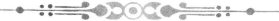

6. Allow the paper to burn completely in the flame of the candle, and then extinguish the candle.

7. Anoint the white candle with lavender oil and light it. Hold the small jar in your hand and say the following incantation: "By the light of this flame, I call upon the forces of the universe to capture the eternal flame of love and devotion ignited in the heart of (name of desired person). May this flame burn brightly forevermore and bind us together in eternal devotion."

8. Allow the white candle to burn down completely, and then extinguish it. Place the ashes of the parchment paper in the small jar and seal it tightly with the lid. Keep the jar in a safe place where it won't be disturbed.

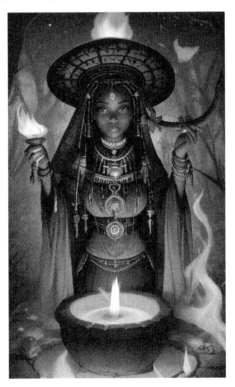

HONEY SWEET LOVE SPELL

The Honey Sweet Love Spell has been passed down through generations of voodoo practitioners. It is said that the spell was first created by a powerful voodoo priestess who used it to win the love of a man who had been unattainable to her for years.

Legend has it that the voodoo priestess was deeply in love with a man who did not return her affections. She tried everything she could think of to win his heart, but nothing worked. In desperation, she turned to her voodoo magic and created the Honey Sweet Love Spell.

The priestess gathered the necessary ingredients and performed the spell with great care and concentration. To her amazement, the man she loved soon began to show interest in her, and within a few weeks, he had fallen deeply in love with her.

The couple's love was said to be strong and long-lasting, and the Honey Sweet Love Spell became famous throughout the voodoo community as a powerful way to bring true love into one's life.

You will need the following:

- 1 pink candle
- One red rose
- Honey

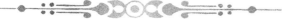

- Small piece of parchment paper
- Red ribbon
- Pen
- A quiet and peaceful room

To perform the spell, follow these steps:

1. Find a quiet and peaceful room to perform the spell. Make sure you will not be disturbed during the ritual.
2. Light the pink candle and place it in front of you.
3. Take the red rose and hold it in your hands. Close your eyes and focus on the scent of the rose. Let the scent fill your senses and relax your mind.
4. While holding the rose, speak the following incantation:
5. "Rose of love, so pure and true, Bring passion and love, anew. With this spell, I do implore, My heart's desire forevermore."
6. Take the parchment paper and write the name of the person you desire on it.
7. Fold the paper in half, with the name facing inward.
8. Dip the rose in the honey and then use it to seal the paper shut.
9. Tie the ribbon around the parchment paper, creating a small bundle.
10. Hold the bundle in your hands and visualize your heart's desire.
11. Speak the following incantation:
    "Honey sweet, this spell I cast, With love and passion, it will last. Bring to me my heart's desire. Let their love burn like a raging fire."
12. Blow out the candle and leave the bundle on your altar. The spell is complete.

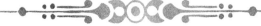

MOONLIGHT RENDEZVOUS SPELL

The Moonlight Rendezvous Spell is a powerful voodoo love spell that is used to bring two people together under the light of the moon. This spell is particularly effective when cast on a full moon night.

The spell is said to have originated in Africa and was brought over to the Caribbean by enslaved people. The power of the full moon was believed to enhance the spell's effectiveness, making it a potent tool for those seeking to unite lovers. However, some caution that the spell should only be used for good intentions and not to force someone into a relationship they do not truly desire, as this can have negative consequences. With the right intentions and a pure heart, the Moonlight Rendezvous Spell can be a powerful tool for bringing together two souls in love.

You will need the following:

- A red candle
- A pink candle
- A white candle
- A small piece of paper
- A pen or pencil
- A moonstone
- A rose quartz crystal
- A piece of red or pink cloth
- Jasmine oil

To perform the spell, follow these steps:

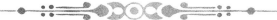

1. Set up your altar by placing the three candles in a triangle formation. The red candle should be at the top, the pink candle on the left, and the white candle on the right.
2. Light the candles and focus your energy on the flames. Take a few deep breaths to ground yourself and center your energy.
3. Write the names of the two people you wish to bring together on the piece of paper. Fold the paper three times and place it in the center of the candle triangle.
4. Take the moonstone and hold it in your left hand. Visualize the two people coming together in love and happiness.
5. Hold the rose quartz crystal in your right hand. Visualize their love growing stronger and more passionate with each passing day.
6. Take a few drops of jasmine oil and anoint the piece of cloth with it. Hold the cloth in both hands and imagine the two people being wrapped in a loving embrace.
7. Place the moonstone and rose quartz crystal on top of the piece of cloth and wrap them up tightly.
8. Place the wrapped bundle in the center of the candle triangle on top of the folded paper.
9. Focus your energy on the flames of the candles and say the following incantation:
   "Under the light of the moon, I call upon the forces of love. Bring together these two souls, and let them know the joy of true love. May their passion burn as bright as the candles before me, And may their love grow stronger with each passing day. So mote it be."
10. Allow the candles to burn down completely. Once the candles have burned out, take the wrapped bundle and bury it in the earth.

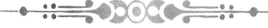

LOVE'S BLOSSOMING GARDEN SPELL

*L*ove's *B*lossoming *G*arden *S*pell is a powerful and enchanting voodoo magic spell that is designed to help you manifest the love and connection you desire in your life. *T*his spell is perfect for anyone looking to attract a new romantic partner, deepen an existing relationship, or rekindle a lost love. *T*he ingredients and incantations used in this spell are all carefully selected to harness the power of nature and the universe to help you achieve your heart's desire.

*S*ome believe the rose petals symbolize love and passion, while the lavender represents purity and healing. *C*hamomile is said to attract love and prosperity, while cinnamon brings warmth and protection. *T*he honey used in the spell is thought to sweeten any potential conflicts or obstacles that may arise in the relationship. *T*his spell has been known to have a powerful and long-lasting effect on those who use it, often leading to the discovery of true love and happiness.

You will need the following:

- Red rose petals
- Lavender buds
- Chamomile flowers
- Cinnamon sticks
- Honey
- Pink or red candles
- A small bowl of water

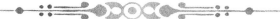

To perform the spell, follow these steps:

1. Begin by gathering all of your ingredients and setting up your sacred space. This can be anywhere that you feel comfortable and free from distractions.
2. Light the candles and place them in a safe spot where they can burn down completely.
3. Combine the rose petals, lavender buds, chamomile flowers, and cinnamon sticks in a bowl.
4. Lightly crush the ingredients together with your fingers, allowing their fragrances to mingle and blend.
5. Take a deep breath and focus your mind on your intentions for this spell.
6. Place the bowl in front of you and pour honey over the top, using a spoon to mix it in with the herbs.
7. With your finger, draw a heart in the honey mixture and say the following incantation: "Love's blossoming garden, hear my plea, Bring me the love that's meant to be. Through the power of this spell, Let my heart and my lover's heart swell."
8. Take a moment to visualize the love you desire and see it manifest in your life.
9. Once you feel ready, light the candles and place the bowl of herbs and honey beside them.
10. Dip your fingers in the water and flick it over the candles, saying: "Water of life, bless this spell. Let my love and my heart be well."
11. Allow the candles to burn down completely, and then dispose of the remaining herbs and honey outside.

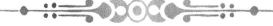

SWEET SERENADE OF LOVE SPELL

The spell is believed to have originated in Africa and was brought over to the Americas during the slave trade. It is said that the spell was often used by women who were seeking to attract the attention of a specific man or to bring a new love into their lives.

Legend has it that the Sweet Serenade of Love Spell was once used by a powerful voodoo priestess, Marie Laveau, who lived in New Orleans in the 19th century. It is said that Marie used the spell to bring together two star-crossed lovers who had been separated by circumstances beyond their control. The spell worked its magic, and the couple was soon reunited in a passionate and long-lasting love affair.

You will need the following:

- A pink or red candle
- A small bottle of rose oil
- A small, decorative bowl filled with honey
- A red rose petal
- A small piece of paper and a pen
- A piece of red string or ribbon
- A small musical instrument (optional)

To perform the spell, follow these steps:

1. Begin by finding a quiet and peaceful space where you can perform the spell without any interruptions. Light the pink or red candle and place it in front of you.
2. Take a few deep breaths and clear your mind. Focus your intention on the spell and the love you wish to attract.
3. Take the small bottle of rose oil and anoint the candle with it. Rub the oil onto the candle in a clockwise motion, focusing your intention on love and desire as you do so.
4. Take the small, decorative bowl filled with honey and dip your finger into it. Take a small amount of honey and place it onto the red rose petal.
5. Write the name of the person you wish to attract on the small piece of paper using the pen. Be sure to write their name in full and with clear intention.
6. Place the red rose petal with the honey onto the piece of paper with the name of the person you wish to attract written on it. Fold the paper so that the rose petal and honey are inside, then tie it closed with the red string or ribbon.
7. Hold the small bundle in your hands and recite the following incantation:
8. "Sweet serenade of love, Bring me the one I'm dreaming of. With this rose and honey so sweet, Bring our hearts together to beat."
9. If you have a small musical instrument, such as a flute or guitar, you can play a simple tune while reciting the incantation. This will add to the potency of the spell.
10. Once you have finished the incantation, place the small bundle onto the candle holder next to the candle.
11. Allow the candle to burn down completely, and then dispose of the remains and the small bundle in a natural location.

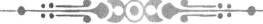

LOVE'S CELESTIAL KISS SPELL

According to legend, the spell was created by a voodoo priestess who wanted to help a couple in her village who were struggling in their relationship. *She* gathered rose petals and lavender oil and chanted a spell under the moonlight to call upon the divine forces for help. *The* couple's love grew stronger after the spell was cast, and they were forever grateful to the voodoo priestess for her magic.

You will need the following:

- A white candle
- A red candle
- Rose petals
- Lavender oil
- A small piece of paper
- A pen or pencil
- A lighter or matches

To perform the spell, follow these steps:

1. Set up a peaceful, romantic environment by lighting some candles and placing rose petals around the room.
2. Take the white candle and carve your initials into it with the pen or pencil. Light the candle and place it in front of you.
3. Take the red candle and carve your partner's initials into it. Light the candle and place it next to the white candle.
4. Take the piece of paper and write your deepest desires for your relationship with your partner. Be specific and make sure to include how you want to feel in the relationship.

5. Anoint the paper with lavender oil and fold it up, holding it tightly in your hand.
6. Visualize the relationship you want with your partner, and feel the love you have for them growing inside of you.
7. Chant the following incantation: "Celestial forces up above, Send me down your divine love. Bring my partner and me closer. Make our bond stronger like no other."
8. Light the folded paper with the flame from the red candle and place it in a fireproof dish.
9. Watch the paper burn, visualizing your desires coming true.
10. Let the candles burn out on their own.

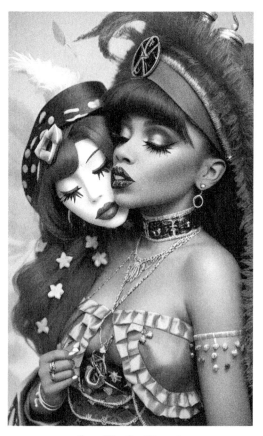

HEARTBEAT SYNCHRONICITY SPELL

The Heartbeat Synchronicity Spell is a powerful voodoo spell that can be used to bring two people closer together and synchronize their heartbeats, creating a deep emotional bond between them. This spell is perfect for couples who are looking to take their relationship to the next level and want to experience a deep connection with their partner.

It is said that the spell was first created by a voodoo priestess who wanted to help two lovers who were separated by distance to feel closer together. She believed that synchronizing their heartbeats would allow them to feel each other's presence even when they were apart. Over time, the spell became more popular and was used by many people to bring them closer to their loved ones. However, it is said that the spell can have unexpected consequences if not performed correctly. Some people have reported feeling a deep emotional bond with someone they did not intend to connect with. It is, therefore important to approach this spell with caution and respect the power of voodoo magic.

You will need the following:

- 2 red candles
- A piece of paper
- A pen or marker
- Rose petals
- 2 lockets

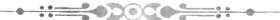

- Red string

To perform the spell, follow these steps:

1. Start by lighting the two red candles and placing them in front of you.
2. On a piece of paper, write the names of the two people who you want to synchronize their heartbeats.
3. Sprinkle rose petals on the paper and fold it in half.
4. Place the paper between the two lockets and tie them together with the red string.
5. Hold the lockets in your hands and close your eyes.
6. Visualize the two people being brought closer together and their heartbeats synchronizing.
7. Recite the following incantation:
   "By the power of the universe, I call upon the spirits to synchronize the heartbeats of [name] and [name]. Let their love be strong and true. Let their hearts beat as one. So mote it be."
8. Hold the lockets close to your heart and blow out the candles.
9. Keep the lockets with you until the spell has taken full effect.

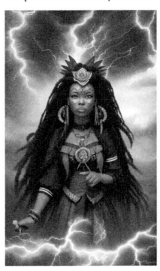

LUSTFUL DESIRES SPELL

The Lustful Desires Spell is a powerful voodoo spell designed to ignite lustful feelings and desires in a specific target.

It was originally used to create intense sexual attraction between two people who were already interested in each other, but over time it has been used for more nefarious purposes. In recent years, voodoo practitioners have warned against using this spell, as it can have uncontrollable effects on the target, leading to stalking, harassment, and even violence. It is important to remember that love and desire should always be consensual, and any spell that promotes non-consensual behavior is unethical and potentially harmful.

You will need the following:

- One red candle
- A picture or personal item of the target
- 3 drops of your own blood
- A lock of your hair
- Red thread
- Red rose petals
- Rose oil
- A small piece of parchment paper
- A pen

To perform the spell, follow these steps:

1. Light the red candle and place it in front of you.
2. Take the picture or personal item of the target and place it on the left side of the candle.
3. Take the parchment paper and the pen and write the target's name on it.
4. Take the lock of your hair and tie it around the parchment paper with the red thread.
5. Add 3 drops of your own blood to the parchment paper and wrap it around the red rose petals.
6. Place the parchment paper and rose petals on the right side of the candle.
7. Anoint the candle with rose oil while visualizing the target being consumed with lustful desires.
8. Light the parchment paper with the candle and let it burn completely, speaking the following:

   "As I light this flame, I call upon the spirits to bring forth the passion and desires of (target's name). May they be consumed with lustful desires for me, and may their heart and soul be filled with longing for my love. So let it be."

9. Let the candle burn down completely.

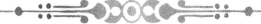

COSMIC LOVE CONNECTION SPELL

Cosmic Love Connection Spell is a powerful and ancient voodoo spell that will connect you with your soulmate in the most profound and intimate way. This spell harnesses the power of the universe to bring two hearts together in a cosmic dance of love.

The spell is an ancient voodoo spell that has been passed down through generations of voodoo practitioners. It is said to have originated in the heart of Africa, where tribal elders used it to connect couples in love.

As the practice of voodoo spread throughout the world, the Cosmic Love Connection Spell became known as one of the most powerful and effective spells for bringing two people together in love. It is believed that the spell works by tapping into the cosmic energy of the universe and aligning it with the intentions of the spellcaster.

There is a legend among voodoo practitioners that tells of a powerful witch doctor who used the Cosmic Love Connection Spell to unite two warring tribes. The spell worked so well that the tribes ended their conflict and joined together as one people. This event is said to have sparked a movement of love and unity that spread throughout the region, bringing peace and prosperity to all who lived there.

You will need the following:

- A red candle
- Rose petals
- Jasmine oil
- A piece of parchment paper
- A pen
- A small bowl of water
- A clear quartz crystal

To perform the spell, follow these steps:

1. Begin by setting your intention. Focus your mind on the person you wish to connect with and visualize your love for them. Think about how you want to feel when you are with them and allow those feelings to fill you up.
2. Light the red candle and place it in front of you. Sprinkle the rose petals around it, forming a circle.
3. Take the parchment paper and write your name and the name of the person you wish to connect with. Draw a heart around the names, and then an infinity symbol over the heart.
4. Anoint the candle with jasmine oil, focusing on your intention and infusing the oil with your desires.
5. Hold the clear quartz crystal in your hand and place it in the bowl of water. Speak the following incantation:
6. "By the power of the universe, I call upon the forces of love. Bring [name of desired person] to me, and connect us in the cosmic dance of love."
7. Hold the parchment paper over the flame of the candle, and let it catch fire. Allow it to burn completely, focusing your intention on the cosmic connection you seek.

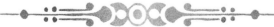

8. Once the parchment paper has burned, take the quartz crystal out of the water and hold it to your heart. Close your eyes and visualize yourself with your soulmate, feeling the love and connection between you.

9. Snuff out the candle and place the crystal on top of the rose petals.

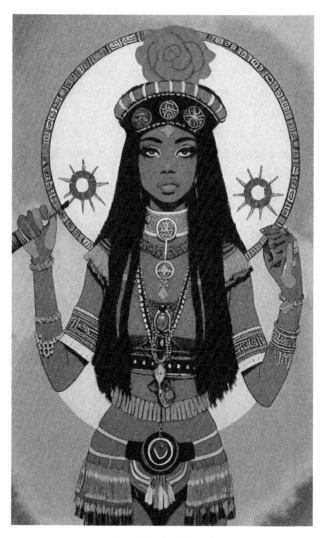

SPELL OF LOVE'S DIVINE INTERVENTION

Spell of Love's Divine Intervention is a powerful voodoo spell that calls upon the divine spirits to bring true love to the caster. This spell is not for the faint of heart and requires a deep connection to the spiritual world.

It is said that the spell was first created by a powerful voodoo priestess who had a deep connection with the spirits and was able to channel their energy to bring about great change.

Legend has it that the priestess was once deeply in love with a man who did not return her affections. Despite her best efforts, he remained oblivious to her feelings and seemed to be moving on with his life. The priestess was heartbroken and turned to the spirits for help.

Through her deep connection with the spiritual world, the priestess was able to create the Spell of Love's Divine Intervention. She performed the spell with great intention and focus, calling upon the spirits to bring her true love, no matter the cost.

Surprisingly, the spell worked, and the man she had been in love with suddenly became deeply enamored with her. However, the love that blossomed between them was not as pure as the priestess had hoped. It was revealed that the man had been under a powerful enchantment that had been placed upon him by

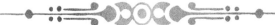

another voodoo practitioner who was jealous of the priestess's power.

The priestess was devastated to learn that her love was not genuine and that she had been manipulated by the spirits. From that day forward, she vowed to use her powers only for good and never again to allow herself to be swayed by the promise of love.

You will need the following:

- Red candle
- Rose petals
- Two small personal items belonging to the caster and the desired partner
- White cloth

To perform the spell, follow these steps:

1. Light the red candle and spread the rose petals around it.
2. Place the two personal items on the white cloth in front of the candle.
3. Focus your energy and intentions on the desired partner.
4. Chant the following incantation three times:
5. "With this candle and these petals, I call upon the divine spirits. Bring forth my true love, my heart's desire. Let us be connected, soul to soul."
6. Blow out the candle and wrap the personal items in the white cloth.
7. Bury the items in the earth, allowing the spirits to carry your message of love to your desired partner.

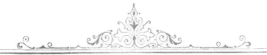

VOODOO WATCHMEN

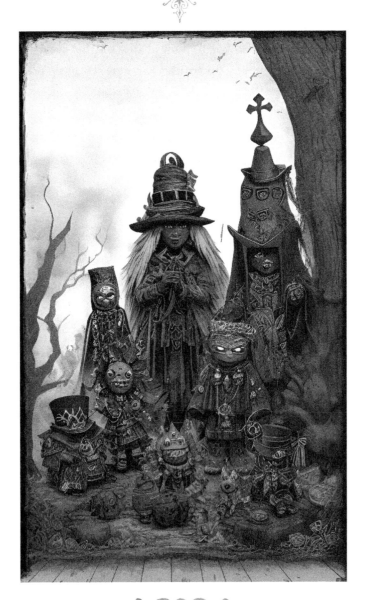

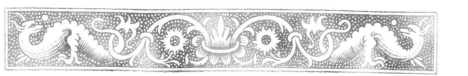

SHADOW SHIELDING SPELL

The Shadow Shielding Spell is a powerful voodoo magic spell that is designed to protect the caster from negative energies and harmful entities. This spell creates a barrier of energy around the caster, which repels any negative influences that may try to penetrate it. It is particularly useful for those who are sensitive to negative energies or who work in environments that are rife with negative influences.

The Shadow Shielding Spell has its roots in the voodoo traditions of West Africa. It is said that the spell was first created by a powerful voodoo priestess who sought to protect herself and her followers from the harmful influences of negative spirits and malevolent entities. Over time, the spell evolved and was passed down from generation to generation, with each new practitioner adding their own unique touch to the incantation and ritual.

Legend has it that one particular voodoo priestess could use the Shadow Shielding Spell to protect an entire village from an army of malevolent spirits bent on destruction. The priestess is said to have stood at the edge of the village, calling forth the shield of black energy, and watched as the spirits bounced off the shield and retreated into the darkness.

You will need the following:

- Black candle

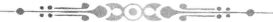

- Protection oil (lavender oil or black pepper oil)
- Salt
- Incense (frankincense or sage)

To perform the spell, follow these steps:

1. Begin by cleansing the area where you will perform the spell. This can be done by smudging with sage or frankincense incense, sprinkling salt around the perimeter of the area, or both.
2. Anoint the black candle with protection oil, starting at the bottom and working your way up to the wick.
3. Light the black candle and place it in front of you.
4. Sit or stand with your feet firmly planted on the ground and take a few deep breaths to center yourself.
5. Visualize a sphere of white light surrounding you. See the light becoming stronger and brighter, and feel it filling you with a sense of peace and protection.
6. Repeat the following incantation three times:
7. "By the power of the divine, I call forth a shield divine. A wall of light around me now, protects me from all harm and ill will."
8. Hold your hands up and visualize a shield of black energy forming around you. See it growing stronger and more impenetrable with each passing moment.
9. When you feel that the shield is strong enough, blow out the candle and give thanks to the spirits for their protection.

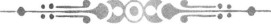

EVIL EYE CHARM

The Evil Eye charm, a powerful spell used to protect oneself from the negative energy and ill wishes of others. This spell is designed to redirect the negative energy back to its source, creating a powerful barrier of protection.

The charm was typically cast on an object, such as a piece of jewelry or a charm, which would serve as a talisman of protection. However, the modern version of the spell involves using a jar or bottle to trap the negative energy and return it to its source.

There is a popular Voodoo legend about the origin of the Evil Eye. According to the legend, a young woman was cursed with the evil eye by a jealous neighbor who coveted her beauty and success. The curse caused the woman to become ill and suffer misfortune, until she sought the help of a Voodoo priestess. The priestess cast a powerful charm that not only protected the woman from the negative energy of her neighbor, but also caused the neighbor to suffer misfortune instead.

You will need the following:

- Small jar or bottle with a lid
- Black ribbon
- Black tourmaline crystal
- Black salt
- Small piece of paper
- Black ink pen

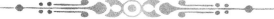

- White candle
- Sage bundle

To perform the spell, follow these steps:

1. Begin by cleansing your space with sage, clearing out any negative energy and setting the intention for the spell. Light the white candle and let it burn throughout the spell.
2. Take the small piece of paper and write the name of the person or people who have been sending negative energy your way. Use black ink and write their name three times.
3. Sprinkle the black salt onto the paper and fold it three times, sealing it with the black ribbon. Place it into the jar or bottle.
4. Hold the black tourmaline crystal in your hand and visualize a protective shield forming around you. Focus on the negative energy bouncing off of the shield and returning to its source.
5. Place the crystal into the jar or bottle with the paper.
6. Close the lid and shake the jar or bottle, visualizing the negative energy being trapped inside and unable to harm you.
7. Hold the jar or bottle in your hands and recite the following incantation:

    "By the power of the Voodoo spirits, I call upon the energy of protection. May this hex send back the negative energy and ill wishes of those who seek to harm me. Let this jar serve as a barrier of protection, trapping the negative energy and preventing it from reaching me. So it be."

8. When you are finished, blow out the white candle and bury the jar or bottle in a safe place, away from your home.

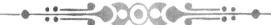

BANSHEE'S BARRIER SPELL

The Banshee's Barrier Spell is a powerful protection spell that summons the spirit of the Banshee to create a barrier of protection around the caster. This spell is particularly useful for protection against harmful spirits and negative energies.

The Banshee is a spirit from Irish folklore who is said to warn of impending death by letting out a blood-curdling scream. The Banshee is also known for her ability to protect those who are worthy of her help. It is said that when a voodoo practitioner invokes the spirit of the Banshee, she will appear and create a barrier of protection around them, shielding them from harm. However, there is a twist to this story. Legend has it that the Banshee will only protect those who have shown kindness and compassion to others. If you have not lived a life of virtue, the Banshee will refuse to help you, and you will be left to fend for yourself against the world's dark forces.

You will need the following:

- A small white candle
- A small black candle
- Sage or palo santo
- Salt
- A small piece of amethyst or black tourmaline
- A feather

To perform the spell, follow these steps:

1. Begin by lighting the white candle and saying the following incantation:

   "Great spirits of light and love, I call upon thee from above. Protect me with your holy might, And banish all darkness from my sight."

2. Light the black candle and place it on your right side.
3. Light the sage or palo santo and cleanse the space around you.
4. Sprinkle a circle of salt around you for protection.
5. Hold the amethyst or black tourmaline in your left hand and the feather in your right hand.
6. Close your eyes and envision a white light surrounding you, protecting you from all harm.
7. Visualize the spirit of the Banshee appearing before you, holding a silver shield.
8. Say the following incantation:

   "Banshee of the misty hills, Protector of the ancient rills. With your shield so bright and true, Protect me from all harm and danger too."

9. Take the feather and use it to draw a circle around you.
10. Blow out the white candle, and let the black candle burn out on its own.
11. Keep the amethyst or black tourmaline on you for added protection.

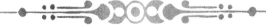

DARK GUARDIAN INVOCATION SPELL

The Dark Guardian Invocation Spell is a powerful voodoo magic spell that is designed to summon and empower a dark guardian spirit to serve as a protector and ally. This spell is particularly useful for those who seek protection from negative energies, dark forces, or malevolent spirits.

The Dark Guardian Invocation Spell is rooted in Haiti's voodoo traditions and the African diaspora. Practitioners originally used it to call upon the spirits of their ancestors and other protective deities to aid them in times of need.

Over time, the spell evolved to incorporate darker, more powerful spirits that could be called upon to protect against malevolent forces. In some cases, practitioners would even seek out the assistance of spirits that were known to be dangerous or unpredictable, believing that their power could be harnessed for good.

You will need the following:

- A black candle
- Dragon's blood incense
- A black obsidian stone
- A black cloth
- Salt
- A black feather
- A small jar of graveyard dirt

To perform the spell, follow these steps:

1. Begin by casting a circle of protection around yourself using salt. This will create a sacred space for you to perform the spell.
2. Light the black candle and the dragon's blood incense. Place the black obsidian stone on the black cloth in front of you.
3. Take the black feather and use it to draw a circle around the stone, moving clockwise. Visualize a protective barrier forming around the stone.
4. Sprinkle a pinch of graveyard dirt onto the stone, and then place the jar of graveyard dirt next to it.
5. Hold your hands over the stone and the jar, and focus your energy on summoning a dark guardian spirit to serve as your protector and ally. Visualize the spirit coming forth from the jar and filling the space around you with its power.
6. Recite the following incantation:

   "By the power of the darkened sky, I summon thee, spirit of the night. Guard and protect me from all harm, with your strength and your might."

7. Allow the candle and incense to burn down completely, and then bury the remains in the jar of graveyard dirt. Place the stone and feather in a safe place where they will not be disturbed.
8. Close the circle of protection by thanking the spirits and releasing them.

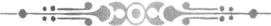

SPIRIT SENTINEL INVOCATION SPELL

Spirit Sentinel Invocation Spell is a powerful Vaudou magic spell that calls upon the spirits to protect and defend the caster against any negative energy or harm. This spell is particularly useful for those who feel vulnerable or under attack, and it can be performed alone or with a group of practitioners.

Legend has it that the Spirit Sentinel Invocation Spell was first created by a powerful Vaudou priestess who lived in the heart of the New Orleans bayou. She was known for her fierce protection spells and her ability to call upon the spirits for help.

One day, a group of bandits came to her village, intent on causing harm and destruction. The priestess knew that she had to act fast to protect her people, so she called upon the spirits to help her.

She performed a powerful ritual, invoking the spirits to protect her and her people. The spirits answered her call, forming a protective shield around the village that kept the bandits at bay.

The bandits were so impressed by the power of the priestess that they decided to leave the village alone and never return. From that day on, the Spirit Sentinel Invocation Spell became a powerful tool for Vaudou practitioners needing protection and defense against harm.

You will need the following:

- A white candle
- A piece of paper
- A pen or pencil
- Sage or other cleansing herbs
- A bowl of salt
- A bowl of water
- An offering for the spirits, such as flowers or fruit

To perform the spell, follow these steps:

1. Find a quiet, peaceful place where you can perform the spell without any distractions.
2. Light the white candle and set it in front of you.
3. Write your intention on the piece of paper, such as "I call upon the spirits to protect me from harm."
4. Hold the paper in your hands and focus on your intention. Visualize a circle of white light forming around you, protecting you from any harm.
5. Place the paper under the candle and sprinkle some sage or other cleansing herbs around the candle.
6. Sprinkle some salt around the candle and place the bowl of salt next to the candle.
7. Sprinkle some water around the candle and place the bowl of water next to the candle.
8. Offer the flowers or fruit to the spirits and ask them to protect you from harm.
9. Close your eyes and recite the following incantation:

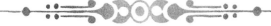

"Spirits of the earth, air, fire, and water, Hear my call and come to my aid. Protect me from all harm and negative energy. Surround me with your divine light and keep me safe."

10. Visualize the spirits surrounding you and forming a protective shield around you.
11. Sit in silence for a few moments, feeling the energy of the spell surround you.
12. When you feel ready, extinguish the candle and dispose of the offering in a natural place.

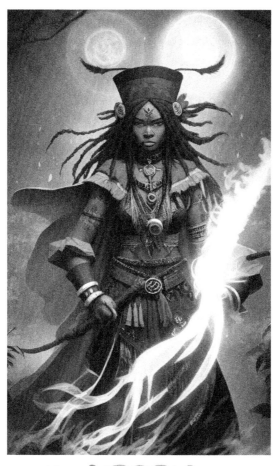

THUNDERBOLT TALISMAN SPELL

The Thunderbolt Talisman Spell is a powerful voodoo spell that imbues an object with the power of thunder and lightning.

The spell has its roots in the mythology of the Haitian Vodou religion, where thunder and lightning were seen as powerful and awe-inspiring forces of nature. The spell was originally developed by a group of powerful voodoo practitioners known as the "Storm Makers," who believed that by harnessing the power of thunder and lightning, they could imbue objects with immense power and energy.

Legend has it that with the talisman charged and ready, the user can wear it to gain its protective powers. The Thunderbolt Talisman Spell provides a powerful shield against physical and magical attacks, and it enhances the wearer's strength and agility.

You will need the following:

- A small piece of copper
- A small piece of iron
- A piece of black cloth
- A small thunderbolt-shaped charm or pendant
- A small piece of parchment paper
- A red marker or pen
- A piece of string or cord
- A thunderstorm (or a recording of thunder)

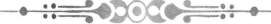

To perform the spell, follow these steps:

1. Begin by finding a quiet and secluded space where you can perform the spell undisturbed. Set up all of your ingredients in front of you.
2. Take the piece of copper and the piece of iron and hold them in your hands. Close your eyes and visualize a powerful thunderstorm raging around you. Focus your energy and intention into the two pieces of metal.
3. Place the copper and iron on the piece of parchment paper. Use the red marker or pen to draw the symbol of thunder on the paper, along with any other symbols or words that feel relevant to you.
4. Fold the paper in half so that the metal pieces are inside, and tie it up with the string or cord. Hold the bundle in your hands and speak the following incantation:

   "Thunder and lightning, hear my call. In this talisman, let your power fall. With each strike and every boom, Grant this object the power of doom."

5. Place the bundle inside the piece of black cloth, and tie it up tightly with the string or cord. Hold the bundle in your hands and visualize the power of thunder and lightning infusing it.
6. Take the thunderbolt charm or pendant and hold it in your hands. Visualize it glowing with a bright and powerful light, and feel its energy pulsing through your body.
7. Speak the following incantation while holding the charm or pendant:

   "Thunder and lightning, hear my plea. Infuse this talisman with energy. With each crack and every flash, Grant this object a powerful smash."

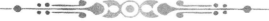

8. Take the charm or pendant and place it inside the black cloth bundle on top of the parchment paper. Hold the bundle in your hands and visualize the energy of thunder and lightning coursing through it.

9. Wait until you hear the sound of thunder or a recording of thunder. At that moment, speak the following incantation:
"Thunder and lightning, it is done. With your power, this spell has won. Let this talisman be infused. With your might, let it be fused."

10. Hold the bundle in your hands and feel the power of thunder and lightning pulsing through it. Please place it in a safe place where it will not be disturbed or touched.

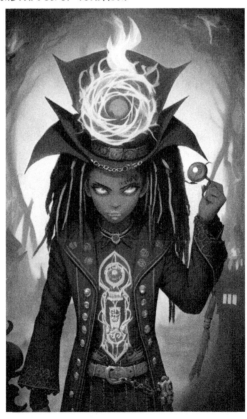

GHOSTLY GUARDIAN CHARM SPELL

The Ghostly Guardian Charm Spell is a powerful voodoo magic that calls forth a spirit to serve as a protective guardian for the caster. This spell is particularly useful for those who seek to protect themselves or their loved ones from harm, evil spirits, or negative energy. The charm works by summoning a ghostly guardian that will stay with the caster and ward off any harmful energies or entities that may come their way

Voodoo practitioners have used the Ghostly Guardian Charm Spell for centuries. According to voodoo tradition, the spell was originally created by a powerful priestess who sought to protect her village from invaders. She called upon a loyal spirit to protect her people and created the charm to ensure the spirit would always remain with them. The spell was passed down from generation to generation and has since been used to protect individuals and families from harm. It is said that the ghostly guardian created by this spell is so strong and so loyal that it will stay with the caster for their entire life, always watching over them and their loved ones. However, there is a dark twist to this spell. Legend has it that if the caster ever breaks their bond with their ghostly guardian, the spirit will turn on them and become their worst nightmare, haunting them until they meet their end. So it is important to remember that the bond between the caster and the guardian is a sacred one that should never be broken.

You will need the following:

- One small bag made of white linen
- One small piece of quartz crystal
- One small piece of black tourmaline
- One small piece of white sage
- One white candle
- A handful of sea salt
- One white feather
- One piece of black string
- 1 photo of the person you wish to protect

To perform the spell, follow these steps:

1. Find a quiet, secluded place where you can cast your spell undisturbed.
2. Light the white candle and sprinkle some sea salt around it to create a protective circle.
3. Take the piece of white sage and light it, letting the smoke fill the circle.
4. Take the quartz crystal and hold it in your left hand. Close your eyes and visualize a protective spirit taking shape around you. Imagine this spirit as a warrior, fierce and loyal.
5. Place the quartz crystal in the white linen bag.
6. Take the black tourmaline and hold it in your right hand. Call upon the spirit world to send you a guardian to protect you and those you love. Ask for a powerful spirit that will serve as your loyal guardian and protector.
7. Place the black tourmaline in the white linen bag.
8. Take the photo of the person you wish to protect and place it in the bag.
9. Tie the bag with the black string and hold it close to your heart.

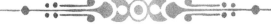

10. Take the white feather and wave it over the bag three times, saying the following incantation:

    "Guardian spirit, hear my call. Protect me and mine from harm's dark thrall With this charm, your power I seek Be my shield, be strong, and be sleek May your loyalty never falter May your protection never alter With your strength, I cast this spell So mote it be, and all is well."

11. Blow out the candle and bury the bag somewhere safe and secret.

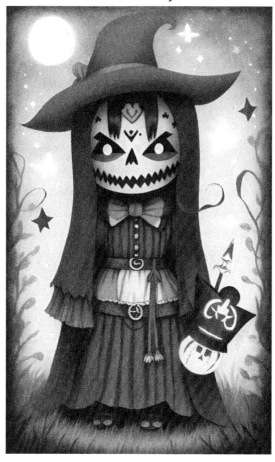

GARGOYLE GUARDIAN INCANTATION SPELL

Gargoyle Guardian Incantation Spell is a powerful voodoo magic spell that calls upon the protection of stone gargoyles.

The spell has its roots in ancient voodoo traditions, where stone gargoyles were believed to possess powerful protective energies. The spell was passed down from generation to generation, with each practitioner adding their own unique variations and enhancements to the ritual. Over time, the spell became one of the most powerful forms of voodoo magic for protection, with its ability to call upon the strength and power of the gargoyle guardians. However, there is a twist to this spell. Some practitioners believe that the spell has a darker side and that the gargoyle may demand a sacrifice in exchange for protection. It is said that those who perform the spell must be cautious lest they fall under the watchful eye of a vengeful gargoyle. As with all forms of voodoo magic, the Gargoyle Guardian Incantation Spell is a potent but unpredictable force capable of great good or great harm, depending on the practitioner's intentions.

You will need the following:

- A small statue or figurine of a gargoyle made of stone or a similar material
- A white candle
- A piece of black cloth or fabric
- A small piece of amethyst crystal

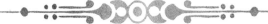

- A handful of dried mugwort
- A small amount of dragon's blood resin
- A cauldron or heat-resistant bowl
- Matches or a lighter

To perform the spell, follow these steps:

1. Set up your working space with all of the necessary ingredients. Make sure the area is clean and free from any distractions.
2. Light the white candle and place it in front of you.
3. Take the black cloth and place the gargoyle statue on top of it.
4. Sprinkle the mugwort and dragon's blood resin over the statue.
5. Hold the amethyst crystal in your hand and recite the following incantation:
6. "Gargoyles of stone and power divine, Protect this space with your ancient design. Let your presence be known, let your strength be felt, Guard this place and those within, let no harm be dealt."
7. Place the amethyst crystal on top of the gargoyle statue.
8. Light the dried herbs on fire and let them burn in the cauldron or bowl.
9. As the smoke rises, recite the following incantation: "Smoke and flame, power of the divine, Cleanse and protect this space, make it mine. Gargoyle guardians, heed my call, Protect me from harm, protect me from all."
10. Hold your hands over the gargoyle statue and visualize it coming to life, its stone body crackling with energy.
11. Place the statue and amethyst crystal in a prominent location in your home or workspace, where it can act as a powerful protector.

VAMPIRE'S BANE BLESSING SPELL

The Vampire's Bane Blessing Spell is a powerful Vaudou spell that is used to ward off vampires and protect the caster from their attacks. This spell is not to be taken lightly, as it requires a deep understanding of the dark arts and a strong will to control its power.

Legend has it that the Vampire's Bane Blessing Spell was first created by a powerful Vaudou priestess who lived deep in the heart of the Louisiana bayou. She was known throughout the land for her mastery of the dark arts, and it was said that she could summon spirits and control the elements with a mere flick of her wrist.

One night, a group of travelers came to the priestess seeking her help. They had been attacked by a pack of vampires and were desperate for a way to protect themselves from further harm. The priestess took pity on them and spent many long hours crafting the Vampire's Bane Blessing Spell.

The travelers followed the priestess's instructions to the letter and were amazed at the power of the spell. Not only were they protected from the vampires, but they also felt a newfound sense of strength and confidence that stayed with them long after they left the bayou.

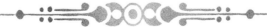

*W*ord of the spell quickly spread throughout the land, and many sought out the priestess's help in creating their own charms and talismans. Some even went so far as to claim that they had seen the priestess herself, walking through the swamp at night with a pack of gargoyles at her side.

You will need the following:

- Fresh garlic cloves
- A silver cross or pendant
- Salt
- Holy water
- Black candle
- Small black bag or pouch
- A drop of the caster's blood

To perform the spell, follow these steps:

1. Begin by purifying your space with the holy water. Sprinkle it around the room and on the items, you will be using in the spell.
2. Light the black candle and place it in front of you.
3. Take the fresh garlic cloves and crush them in your hands. Visualize their potent smell and power, warding off any vampires or dark spirits.
4. Sprinkle a small amount of salt on the garlic, and hold it up to the flame of the black candle. As you do so, recite the following incantation:
   "Vampire's Bane, protect me now, With garlic, salt, and silver vow. Turn away the fangs of death. With this spell, I shall be blessed."
5. Take the silver cross or pendant and hold it up to the flame of the black candle. Recite the following incantation:

"Silver cross, of holy light, Protect me from the vampire's bite.
With your power, guard me well, And cast the darkness back to
hell."

6. Take the small black bag or pouch and place the garlic, salt, and
   silver cross or pendant inside. Add a drop of your own blood, and
   sprinkle a few drops of holy water on top.
7. Tie the bag shut, and hold it up to the flame of the black candle.
   Recite the following incantation:
   "Vampire's Bane, with blood and might, Protect me now both day
   and night. With this charm, I am made whole, And shielded from
   the vampire's toll."
8. Blow out the black candle, and place the bag or pouch in a safe
   place where it will not be disturbed. The spell is now complete.

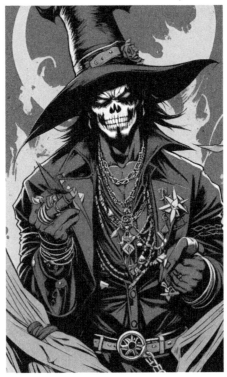

ENCHANTED EYE PROTECTION SPELL

Enchanted Eye Protection Spell! A powerful and ancient Voodoo ritual that has been passed down through generations of practitioners. This spell is designed to protect the eyes of the caster from any harm, including physical, spiritual, and emotional damage.

The Enchanted Eye Protection Spell is said to have originated in West Africa, where Voodoo practitioners used it to protect their eyes from harm during spiritual ceremonies. The spell was later brought to the New World by enslaved Africans, where it became an important part of Voodoo practice.

However, there is a twist to the history of this spell. Legend has it that the Enchanted Eye Protection Spell was created by a powerful Voodoo priestess who had the ability to see into the future. The priestess foresaw a time when Voodoo would be outlawed and its practitioners persecuted. She created the spell as a way to protect future generations of Voodoo practitioners from harm, both physical and spiritual.

You will need the following:

- A small bag made of red fabric
- A pinch of salt
- Three bay leaves
- One teaspoon of black pepper

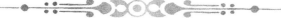

- One teaspoon of dried rosemary
- One teaspoon of dried thyme
- One teaspoon of dried basil
- One small piece of ginger root
- One small piece of garlic
- One small piece of onion
- One small piece of lodestone

To perform the spell, follow these steps:

1. Begin by lighting a black candle, and placing it in front of you. This will help to ward off any negative energy during the spell.
2. Take the small bag made of red fabric, and place it in front of you.
3. Add a pinch of salt to the bag, followed by the three bay leaves.
4. Next, add the black pepper, dried rosemary, dried thyme, and dried basil to the bag. Make sure to mix the ingredients together thoroughly.
5. Take the small piece of ginger root, garlic, and onion, and place them in the bag.
6. Finally, add the small piece of lodestone to the bag. This will help to strengthen the spell and provide additional protection.
7. Once all the ingredients are in the bag, close it tightly and hold it in your hands.
8. Focus your mind on the bag and chant the following incantation: "By the power of the spirits and the magic of Voodoo, I call upon thee to protect my eyes from harm. Let no harm come to me, physically, emotionally, or spiritually, As I walk my path in this world."
9. Chant the incantation three times while visualizing a white protective light surrounding your eyes.
10. Once you have completed the incantation, open your eyes and blow out the candle.

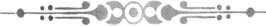

CURSE REVERSAL CHARM

The Curse Reversal Charm is a powerful Vaudou charm used to undo curses and hexes that have been placed on individuals or objects. This charm requires specific ingredients and the use of powerful incantations to successfully remove the effects of a curse.

Legend has it that the Curse Reversal Charm was created by the powerful voodoo priestess Marie Laveau. The story goes that a young woman came to her seeking help after she was cursed by a jealous rival. Marie Laveau knew that the curse was very powerful, but she also knew that she had the knowledge and power to reverse it.

She gathered the ingredients for the charm and cast the spell on behalf of the young woman. The spell was so powerful that it broke the curse and reversed it, causing the person who had placed the curse to experience the effects of their own negative energy.

Since then, the Curse Reversal Charm has become one of the most powerful spells in the voodoo tradition, used by practitioners to break curses and hexes and to protect against negative energy. The charm is considered to be so effective that it is believed to have the power to reverse even the most powerful curses, no matter how long they have been in place.

You will need the following:

- White candle
- Black salt
- Fresh basil leaves
- Dried rosemary
- Dried thyme
- Dried lavender
- A piece of paper
- Pen or pencil
- Red string or cord

To perform the charm, follow these steps:

1. Light the white candle and place it in front of you.
2. Mix the black salt, basil, rosemary, thyme, and lavender together in a bowl.
3. On the piece of paper, write the name of the person or object that has been cursed.
4. Sprinkle the mixture of herbs over the name.
5. Fold the paper three times towards you and tie it with the red string or cord.
6. Hold the bundle of paper over the flame of the white candle and say the following incantation: "By the power of the spirits, I break this curse. Let the energies be released, and the curse be reversed."
7. Burn the paper in the flame of the candle and let it burn completely.
8. As the paper burns, say the incantation one more time.
9. Extinguish the candle and bury the ashes of the paper in the ground.

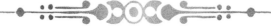

SERAPHIC SHIELD INVOCATION

The Seraphic Shield Invocation spell is a powerful Vaudou magic spell that is believed to summon the protection of the holy Seraphim. This spell requires a skilled practitioner to cast it and several potent ingredients to make it work.

According to ancient Vaudou lore, the spell was first created by a powerful voodoo priestess named Adina. She was known throughout the land for her mastery of the dark arts and her ability to summon powerful spirits to do her bidding.

One day, Adina was approached by a young woman who was being stalked by a dangerous predator. The woman begged Adina for help and agreed to cast a spell to protect her. Drawing on her knowledge of the ancient texts, Adina created the Seraphic Shield Invocation spell.

The spell worked perfectly, and the young woman was never harmed. News of Adina's spell spread quickly, and soon many people were seeking her out for protection. Adina became known as the protector of the people, and her spell was used for generations to keep the community safe.

However, one day Adina's spell went horribly wrong. A group of bandits, seeking to loot the village, attacked Adina's temple. In the chaos of the battle, Adina was killed, and her spellbook was lost. The villagers believed that Adina's magic

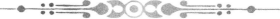

had died with her, and they were left defenseless against their enemies.

Years later, a young priestess discovered Adina's lost spellbook. She studied it carefully and eventually found the Seraphic Shield Invocation spell. Realizing the power of the spell, she began using it to protect her people. Word of the spell spread once again, and it became one of the most sought-after spells in all of Vaudou's magic. And so, the legacy of Adina and her powerful Seraphic Shield Invocation spell lived on, protecting generations of Vaudou practitioners from harm.

You will need the following:

- A white candle
- Angelica root
- Basil
- Eucalyptus
- Frankincense
- Myrrh
- Patchouli oil
- Sandalwood incense
- White sage

To perform the spell, follow these steps:

1. Light the white candle and the sandalwood incense.
2. Sprinkle angelica root, basil, eucalyptus, and frankincense around the candle.

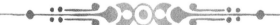

3. Rub patchouli oil on your forehead, wrists, and the bottoms of your feet.
4. Burn the white sage and walk through the smoke to purify your aura.
5. Stand before the candle and close your eyes. Focus on the flame and breathe deeply.
6. Recite the following incantation: "Seraphim, come to my aid. Shield me from all harm and danger. Surround me with your holy light and keep me safe from all evil."
7. Picture a brilliant white light surrounding you like a shield.
8. Visualize the Seraphim standing guard around you, and their wings spread out to protect you.
9. Hold this image for as long as you can. When you are ready, blow out the candle and end the spell.

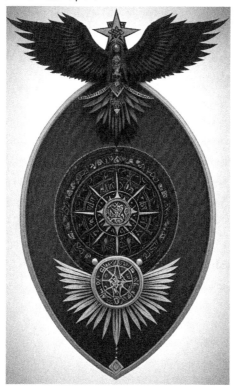

SPIRIT ANCHOR SPELL

The Spirit Anchor Spell is a powerful voodoo spell that allows the caster to bind the spirit of a person or object to a physical anchor, making it impossible for the spirit to leave. This spell can be used to keep spirits trapped in a particular location, prevent them from possessing other bodies, or to keep them from causing harm.

Legend has it that the Spirit Anchor Spell was first created by a powerful voodoo priestess who lived in the swamps of Louisiana. She used the spell to keep the spirits of her enemies trapped in her lair, preventing them from causing harm to her or her followers. Over time, the spell became a popular tool among voodoo practitioners, who used it to trap all manner of spirits and entities.

However, the spell also had a dark side. Some voodoo priests and priestesses began to use it to trap the spirits of innocent people, keeping them as slaves or using them for their own nefarious purposes. It was said that the anchor would become cursed, drawing the target's spirit down into the depths of hell itself.

The Spirit Anchor Spell requires several ingredients and a great deal of focus and concentration, but the results are well worth the effort.

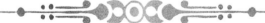

You will need the following:

- A small anchor made of iron
- A vial of graveyard dirt
- A black candle
- A red candle
- A white candle
- A piece of cloth to wrap the anchor
- A strand of the target's hair
- A personal item belonging to the target
- A cauldron or fire-safe container
- Charcoal briquettes
- Salt
- Holy water
- A bell

To perform the spell, follow these steps:

1. Set up your ritual space by laying out your materials and lighting the charcoal briquettes in your cauldron or fire-safe container.
2. Light the black candle and call upon the spirits of the dead to aid you in your spellcasting.
3. Take the strand of the target's hair and wrap it around the anchor, tying it tightly in place.
4. Sprinkle the graveyard dirt over the anchor and recite the incantation: "Spirits of the dead, hear my plea, Bind this spirit to this anchor for eternity, Let it never leave, let it never roam, Let it be trapped, let it be alone."
5. Light the red candle and hold the personal item belonging to the target in your hands. Close your eyes and focus your energy on the item, visualizing the spirit of the target being drawn into it.
6. Place the personal item on the cloth and wrap it tightly around the anchor, securing it in place.

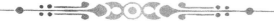

7. Light the white candle and sprinkle salt over the cloth-wrapped anchor, saying: "Salt of the earth, purify and protect, Keep this spirit bound, never to defect."
8. Sprinkle holy water over the anchor and ring the bell three times.
9. Close the ritual by thanking the spirits and snuffing out the candles.

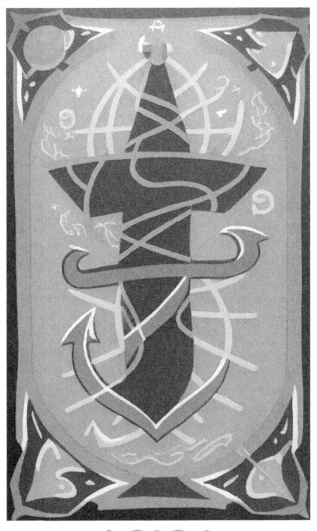

DARK MAGIC DETERRENT SPELL

The Dark Magic Deterrent Spell is a powerful ritual that can protect you from negative energies and dark forces. It requires a few rare and exotic ingredients, a strong will, and the right incantations.

Legend has it that the Dark Magic Deterrent Spell was first created by a powerful Voodoo priestess who lived in the deep forests of Haiti. Her name was Marie Laveau, and she was revered by the locals as a healer and a protector. Marie Laveau had a deep understanding of the spiritual world and knew how to use magic to help those in need.

One day, a dark sorcerer came to her, seeking her help in performing a forbidden ritual. The sorcerer was intent on using black magic to gain power and control over others. But Marie Laveau knew the dangers of such magic and refused to help him.

Enraged, the sorcerer swore vengeance on Marie Laveau and her followers. He began sending evil spirits and negative energies to attack them, but Marie Laveau was not one to be easily defeated. She consulted with the spirits of the ancestors and came up with the Dark Magic Deterrent Spell, a powerful ritual that would protect her and her people from harm.

Marie Laveau performed the ritual with great success, and the sorcerer could never harm her or her followers again.

You will need the following:

- A black candle
- A white candle
- A bowl of sea salt
- A few drops of dragon's blood oil
- A piece of black tourmaline
- A pinch of graveyard dirt
- A piece of chicken bone
- A few strands of your own hair

To perform the spell, follow these steps:

1. Begin by setting up your altar with the black candle on the left and the white candle on the right. Place the bowl of sea salt in the center.
2. Anoint the black candle with dragon's blood oil and sprinkle some graveyard dirt around it. Light the black candle and say the following incantation three times: "By the power of the dark, I call upon the spirits to protect me from harm. Let no evil energy pass through this barrier."
3. Anoint the white candle with dragon's blood oil and sprinkle some sea salt around it. Light the white candle and say the following incantation three times: "By the power of the light, I call upon the spirits to purify this space. Let only positive energy flow through this barrier."

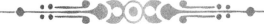

4. Place the black tourmaline in the bowl of sea salt and add a few drops of dragon's blood oil to it. Stir the mixture with the chicken bone while chanting the following incantation three times: "By the power of the elements, I charge this crystal with the strength to banish all negativity."

5. Add a pinch of graveyard dirt and a few strands of your own hair to the mixture. Say the following incantation three times while visualizing a protective shield around you: "By the power of my own spirit, I am shielded from all harm. Let no dark energy penetrate this shield."

6. Finally, take the bowl of sea salt and sprinkle it around the perimeter of your home or the space you wish to protect. Say the following incantation three times: "By the power of the ancestors and the spirits of the earth, I banish all negative energies from this space. Let only peace and harmony prevail."

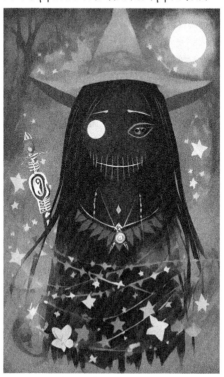

NECROTIC NULLIFICATION SPELL

The Necrotic Nullification Spell is a powerful Vaudou ritual that can neutralize the harmful effects of necromancy magic. This spell is particularly useful against curses, diseases, and other afflictions that are caused by dark magic.

The Necrotic Nullification Spell has a long and storied history in Voodoo magic. According to legend, the spell was first used by a powerful Voodoo queen named Krabba, who lived in New Orleans in the 19th century. Krabba was renowned for her skill in magic, and she was feared by many who believed she possessed the power to control life and death.

One day, Krabba was approached by a wealthy merchant who had fallen under the spell of a rival Voodoo priestess. The merchant begged Krabba to help him, offering her a large sum of money in exchange for her services.

Krabba accepted the merchant's offer and set about casting the Necrotic Nullification Spell. The spell was successful, and the merchant was freed from the spell of the rival priestess. However, Krabba discovered that the spell had unintended consequences. The spell had not only nullified the rival priestess's magic, but it had also nullified her own magic as well. From that day forward, Krabba was never able to cast magic again.

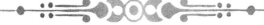

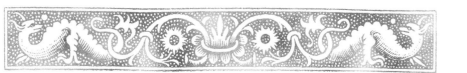

You will need the following:

- A black candle
- A piece of paper with the name of the person or entity to be nullified written in blood
- Salt
- A handful of graveyard dirt
- A small piece of cloth soaked in holy water
- A chicken feather

To perform the spell, follow these steps:

1. Begin by lighting the black candle and placing it in front of you. Sit cross-legged on the ground and hold the piece of paper with the name of the entity you wish to nullify in your hands.
2. Sprinkle a circle of salt around you and place the graveyard dirt in the center of the circle.
3. Recite the following incantation while holding the paper with the name of the entity:
4. "From the grave, I call upon the spirits of the dead To nullify this curse and all that it has fed With this ritual, I break the chains of dark magic And send back to its source, this curse so tragic."
5. Sprinkle a pinch of salt on the piece of paper and then fold it up.
6. Place the folded paper on the graveyard dirt and then light the cloth soaked in holy water on fire.
7. Hold the burning cloth over the paper and let the ashes fall onto the graveyard dirt.
8. Take the chicken feather and use it to stir the ashes and graveyard dirt together while repeating the incantation.
9. Finally, blow out the black candle to complete the ritual.

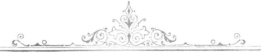

Jinxes and Hexes

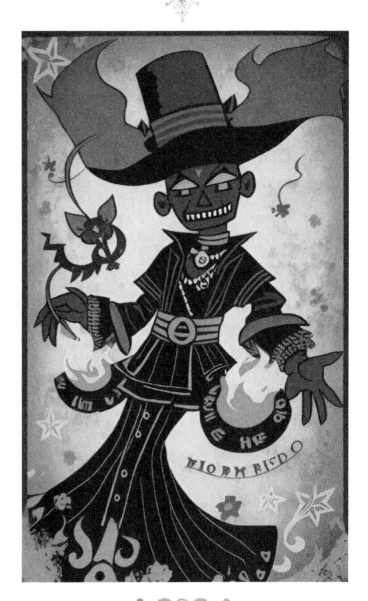

CURSE OF THE BLACK WIDOW

Curse of the Black Widow is a powerful voodoo spell that is said to bring vengeance upon one's enemies. The curse is believed to be named after the deadly spider that devours its mate, just as the victim of this spell is consumed by the curse.

The Curse of the Black Widow has a long and storied history in voodoo culture. Legend has it that the spell was first cast by a powerful voodoo queen who had been betrayed by her lover. Seeking revenge, she summoned the spirits of the dead to aid her in creating the curse.

The voodoo queen gathered the venom of a black widow spider, the skin of a snake, and the salt of the earth and mixed them together in a ritual that lasted three days and three nights. When the curse was complete, she buried the bundle in the ground and waited for her lover's downfall.

Days turned to weeks, and weeks turned to months, but the voodoo queen's lover showed no sign of being affected by the curse. In a fit of rage, the queen dug up the bundle and discovered that it had been replaced with a note that read:

"The only thing more powerful than revenge is forgiveness."

The voodoo queen was struck by the message and realized the error of her ways. She forgave her lover and used her powers to heal rather than harm from that day forward.

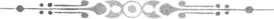

Despite this lesson, the Curse of the Black Widow remains a potent spell in the voodoo tradition and is often used by those seeking retribution. But as with all magic, it is important to remember that what goes around comes around and that forgiveness is a powerful force that can overcome even the strongest of curses.

You will need the following:

- Black widow spider (dead or alive)
- Black candles
- Graveyard dirt
- Snake skin
- Black pepper
- Salt
- Red cloth
- Voodoo doll (optional)

To perform the spell, follow these steps:

1. Begin by creating a circle of protection around yourself using the black candles. Light them and arrange them in a circle, then step inside the circle to begin the spell.
2. Sprinkle the graveyard dirt around the perimeter of the circle to invoke the spirits of the dead. This will add to the power of the spell.
3. Take the black widow spider and crush it in your hands. Make sure to visualize your target as you do this. If you have a voodoo doll of the person, you can also stick the spider to the doll to enhance the spell.

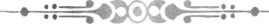

4. Add the snake skin, black pepper, and salt to the crushed spider. Mix them together in your hands while chanting the following incantation:

   "Black widow, weave your web of revenge. Let the venom of the snake poison my enemy's mind. Let the salt cleanse their spirit of all that is good. So mote it be."

5. Once you have finished chanting, spread the mixture onto the red cloth. Wrap the cloth around the voodoo doll (if you have one), or simply tie it into a bundle with string.
6. Take the bundle outside and bury it in the ground, making sure to cover it with dirt. Alternatively, you can throw it into a river to symbolize the washing away of your enemy's good fortune.
7. To seal the spell, chant the following incantation:

   "May the spirits of the dead hear my plea. Let this curse be cast and bring my enemy to their knees. So mote it be."

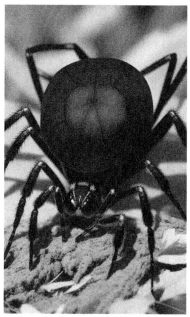

BLOOD MOON HEX

Blood Moon Hex is a powerful Voodoo spell that can be used to bring about change and influence events to achieve a desired outcome. This hex is particularly potent when cast during a Blood Moon, a rare astronomical event that occurs when the Earth casts a reddish shadow on the Moon. The Blood Moon is a time of great power; this hex can harness that energy to bring about powerful results.

The Blood Moon Hex is said to have originated in the early 1800s in New Orleans, Louisiana. According to legend, a powerful Voodoo priestess named Marie Laveau created the spell during a particularly potent Blood Moon. She used the spell to bring about the downfall of a rival Voodoo practitioner who had been spreading lies and rumors about her.

However, there is a twist to this story. Some believe that Marie Laveau didn't create the spell but learned it from a mysterious traveler who passed through the city during the Blood Moon. It is said that this traveler was a practitioner of dark magic and had come to New Orleans to teach Marie Laveau and her followers the secrets of his craft.

You will need the following:

- One red candle
- One black candle
- One Blood Moon stone

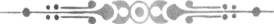

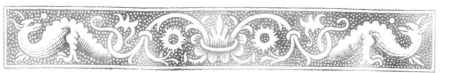

- One vial of bat blood
- One vial of spider venom
- One piece of parchment paper
- One quill pen
- One cauldron
- One wooden spoon

To perform the spell, follow these steps:

1. Begin by lighting the red candle and placing it to your right and the black candle to your left.
2. Take the piece of parchment paper and the quill pen, and write the name of the person or thing you wish to hex.
3. Draw a pentagram on the paper around the name.
4. Place the Blood Moon stone in the center of the pentagram.
5. Pour the bat blood and spider venom into the cauldron.
6. Hold your hands over the cauldron and recite the following incantation: "By the power of the Blood Moon, I call upon the spirits to aid me in this hex. Let the blood of the bat and the venom of the spider be the agents of my will. Let my hex be strong and true, and bring about the change I desire."
7. Take the parchment paper with the name and pentagram, and place it in the cauldron.
8. Stir the mixture with the wooden spoon, while reciting the following incantation: "Blood and venom, fire and ice, let this hex be my sacrifice. Let my will be done, let my desire be met, with this spell I do beset."
9. Take the parchment paper out of the cauldron and let it dry.
10. Once it's dry, light the edges of the parchment paper with the black candle and say: "By the power of the Blood Moon, let this hex take hold. Let my will be done, and the change I desire unfold."

GRAVEYARD BINDING

Graveyard Binding is a powerful Voodoo spell used to bind an individual to a specific location, typically a graveyard. This spell is intended to keep the target bound to the location, preventing them from leaving or causing harm to others.

The Graveyard Binding spell is an ancient Voodoo ritual that dates back centuries. Practitioners commonly used it to keep dangerous individuals from causing harm to their community. However, the spell was often reserved for the most heinous of criminals, as it was believed to be a powerful and irreversible curse.

Legend has it that a powerful Voodoo priestess was once wrongfully accused of a crime and sentenced to death. Before her execution, she cast the Graveyard Binding spell on her accusers, binding them to the cemetery where she was buried. The curse was so powerful that it kept the individuals bound to the graveyard for eternity, their spirits forever trapped in the same location as the priestess who had cursed them.

Over time, the spell became a cautionary tale among Voodoo practitioners, warning of the dangers of using such powerful magic without just cause. To this day, the Graveyard Binding spell is considered one of the most powerful and dangerous spells in the Voodoo tradition.

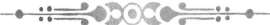

You will need the following:

- Grave dirt from a cemetery
- A black candle
- A photo or personal item of the target
- A piece of paper and pen
- A black thread
- A small black pouch

To perform the spell, follow these steps:

1. Begin by lighting the black candle and placing it in front of you.
2. Take the piece of paper and write the name of the target and their date of birth.
3. Hold the personal item or photo of the target in your hands and focus on their energy.
4. Sprinkle a pinch of grave dirt onto the photo or personal item.
5. Fold the paper and personal item together and tie them with the black thread.
6. Place the bound items into the black pouch.
7. Hold the pouch in your hands and chant the following incantation:

   "By the power of the spirits, I bind you to this place. May you never leave, may you never harm another. May the spirits of this graveyard hold you tight, For as long as I desire, day or night."

8. Once the incantation is complete, place the pouch into the center of the black candle's flame and let it burn.
9. As the candle burns down, visualize the target being bound to the graveyard.
10. Once the candle has burned down completely, bury the ashes and remnants of the pouch in the graveyard.

SHADOW BANISHMENT CURSE

The Shadow Banishment Curse is a powerful voodoo spell used to banish an individual's shadow, rendering them powerless and unable to cause harm. The curse is a last resort, as it requires the use of dark magic and should only be used in extreme situations.

The Shadow Banishment Curse has a long and dark history in voodoo lore. Legend has it that the voodoo queen Boli Shahin first used the curse in New Orleans during the mid-19th century. A wealthy plantation owner had been terrorizing the local community with his cruel and oppressive ways, and Boli was approached by a group of enslaved individuals who begged her for help.

Boli agreed to help but warned the group that the Shadow Banishment Curse was a powerful and dangerous spell and could only be used in extreme situations. The group assured Boli that they were willing to take the risk, and together they performed the curse, banishing the plantation owner's shadow and rendering him powerless.

The curse worked, and the plantation owner was never able to harm anyone again. However, the group who had performed the spell began to experience strange and unsettling occurrences. They reported seeing the plantation owner's shadow following

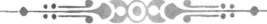

them everywhere they went and hearing his voice whispering in their ears.

Eventually, the group realized that they had inadvertently trapped the plantation owner's shadow inside themselves and were forced to live with the consequences of their actions. From that day forward, the Shadow Banishment Curse was regarded with great caution and respect in voodoo circles and was only used as a last resort when all other options had been exhausted.

You will need the following:

- A black candle
- A white candle
- A voodoo doll or photo of the target
- Salt
- An obsidian or black tourmaline crystal
- A cauldron or heat-proof container
- A black feather
- A piece of paper and a pen

To perform the spell, follow these steps:

1. Cast a protective circle around yourself and your working area, using salt to create a physical barrier.
2. Light the black candle, representing the target's shadow, and the white candle, representing the light that will banish it.
3. Take the voodoo doll or photo of the target and hold it over the cauldron or heat-proof container.
4. Recite the following incantation:

"By the power of the dark and the light, I banish your shadow from sight. No harm will come from your hand, For your shadow is now forever banned."

5. Sprinkle salt over the doll or photo to seal the spell.
6. Place the obsidian or black tourmaline crystal on top of the salt.
7. Write the target's name on the piece of paper and light it with the black candle and speak the words:

"Banish this shadow, banish this curse, Let it be known, let it be heard. With the power of the dark and the light, I banish this shadow from sight."

8. Drop the burning paper into the cauldron or container, using the black feather to stir the ashes until they are completely cooled.
9. Once the ashes are cool, bury them in the ground, ensuring that the target's shadow is forever sealed away.

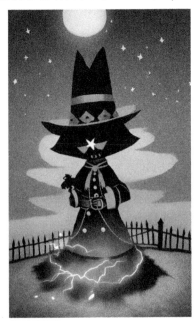

TOXIC TEARS OF THE UNREQUITED HEX

Toxic Tears of the *Unrequited Hex* is a powerful *Voodoo* curse that is used to inflict severe emotional pain on someone who has rejected your love or affection. *This* hex harnesses the power of toxic energy and negative emotions to create a powerful and long-lasting curse.

It is said that it was first used by a powerful *Voodoo* priestess who had been spurned by a lover. *The* hex was so potent that it drove the lover to madness, ultimately leading to his demise. *The* curse is believed to draw its power from the intense emotions of the caster and the target and the rusty nails, which symbolize the pain and suffering caused by the rejection. *It* is said that the curse can only be broken if the caster forgives the target or if the target reciprocates their love. *However,* many believe that the curse is so strong that it can never be lifted, and the toxic tears of the unrequited will forever haunt the target.

You will need the following:

- A small jar with a lid
- Black candles
- Black pepper
- Lemon juice
- Black salt
- 9 rusty nails
- A photo or personal item belonging to the target

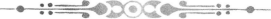

To perform the spell, follow these steps:

1. Begin by lighting the black candles and taking a few deep breaths to center your energy and focus your intent.
2. Take the small jar and add a pinch of black pepper, a few drops of lemon juice, and a pinch of black salt to the bottom of the jar.
3. Take the personal item or photo of the target and place it in the jar, making sure that it is completely covered by the mixture.
4. Take the rusty nails and pierce them through the lid of the jar, making sure that the nails penetrate the photo or personal item inside.
5. Seal the jar with the lid and shake it vigorously while reciting the following incantation: "Toxic tears of unrequited love, Inflict pain from below and above, Blacken their heart and darken their soul, This curse shall take its toll."
6. Once the incantation is complete, blow out the black candles and leave the jar in a dark place where it will not be disturbed.

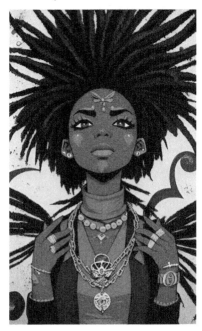

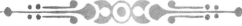

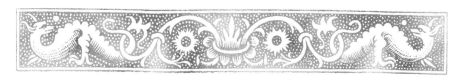

SOUL ERASER HEX

The Soul Eraser Hex is a powerful voodoo spell that is designed to completely erase a person's soul from existence. It is considered one of the most dangerous spells in voodoo magic, as it is believed that once a person's soul is erased, they can never be resurrected or reincarnated.

Once upon a time, in the heart of New Orleans, there lived a powerful voodoo priestess named Marie. She was known throughout the city for her mystical abilities and the unique spells that she could cast. Her magic was feared and respected, and many believed that she had the power to control the very essence of life and death.

Marie was approached by a wealthy businessman named Michael, who had a burning desire to destroy his enemy, a rival businessman named David. Michael had tried every possible means to bring David down but had failed miserably every time. He was now desperate and willing to do anything to ensure that David would never rise again.

Marie listened to Michael's request and pondered for a while before finally agreeing to cast the Soul Eraser Hex on David. Michael handed over a lock of David's hair, and Marie set to work.

She began the ritual by lighting a black candle and placing it in a cauldron. She then wrote David's name on a piece of parchment paper using a black pen and placed his lock of hair on top. She sprinkled some graveyard dirt on the parchment paper and folded it three times before placing it in the cauldron.

Marie chanted the incantation to erase David's soul from existence as the parchment paper burned. But as she finished the spell, something strange happened. The cauldron began to shake, and dark energy burst out of it, enveloping Marie in its embrace.

Marie's eyes rolled back into her head, and she began to convulse violently. Michael, who had been watching from the sidelines, was horrified as he saw Marie's body being consumed by the dark energy. He tried to stop the ritual, but it was too late.

When the energy dissipated, David's lock of hair lay on the floor, untouched. Marie's body lay motionless on the ground, her eyes staring into space. Michael tried to revive her, but she was beyond help.

In a moment of realization, Michael understood what had happened. Marie had not cast the Soul Eraser Hex on David; instead, the spell had backfired, erasing Marie's own soul from existence.

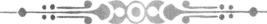

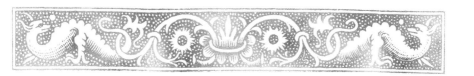

Michael was shaken to the core by what he had witnessed, and he realized that he had been consumed by his own greed and desire for revenge. He had unwittingly caused the death of a powerful and respected voodoo priestess, all for his own selfish reasons.

From that day on, Michael lived the rest of his life in regret, haunted by the memory of Marie's death and the realization that sometimes, the greatest enemy lies within ourselves.

You will need the following:

- A black candle
- A piece of parchment paper
- A black pen
- A lock of hair or personal item from the target
- A graveyard dirt
- A cauldron or fireproof bowl
- A black cloth

To perform the spell, follow these steps:

1. Begin by lighting the black candle and placing it in the cauldron or fireproof bowl.
2. Write the name of the target on the parchment paper using the black pen.
3. Place the lock of hair or personal item from the target on the parchment paper.
4. Sprinkle some graveyard dirt on top of the parchment paper.
5. Fold the parchment paper three times and place it in the cauldron.
6. As the parchment paper burns, recite the following incantation:

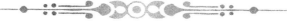

"Soul of [target's name], I erase you from existence, Your soul no longer has persistence. Gone forever from this world, Into darkness, your spirit is hurled."

7. Continue reciting the incantation until the parchment paper has been completely burned to ashes.
8. Once the parchment paper has been burned, extinguish the candle and dispose of the ashes in a place far away from your home.
9. Wrap the remaining materials in the black cloth and bury it in a graveyard or another place associated with death.

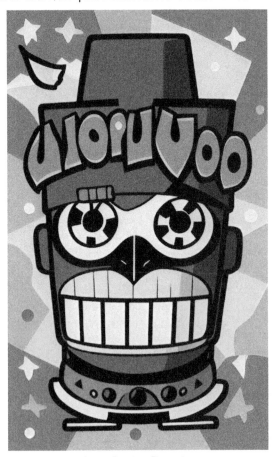

CATACLYSMIC KARMA HEX

The Cataclysmic Karma hex is a powerful spell that brings devastating consequences to the target. It works by using the target's negative energy against them, causing their karma to collapse in on itself and leading to a series of unfortunate events.

It was first created by a powerful Voodoo priestess named Adya Sount'tò. Legend has it that she used the spell to exact revenge on her enemies, causing them to experience a series of unfortunate events that ultimately led to their downfall.

However, the twist in the story is that some believe that Adya Sount'tò did not create the spell at all but instead stole it from a rival priestess. This priestess is said to have cursed Marie and her descendants, causing them to suffer a similar fate as their enemies.

You will need the following:

- A black candle
- A piece of paper
- Black ink
- A personal item from the target
- Graveyard dirt
- A pinch of cayenne pepper
- Salt
- A black pouch

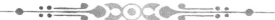

To perform the spell, follow these steps:

1. Light the black candle and focus on the target's negative energy.
2. Write the target's name on the piece of paper using black ink.
3. Sprinkle graveyard dirt on the paper and fold it into a small packet.
4. Add the personal item of the target to the packet.
5. Sprinkle a pinch of cayenne pepper and salt over the packet.
6. Recite the following incantation: "Karma, karma, hear my call, Cataclysmic hex, take hold. Target's energy turned against, Karma collapses, fate incensed. Bring misfortune, bring despair. Let no good luck be theirs to share."
7. Seal the packet in the black pouch and hide it away in a dark place.

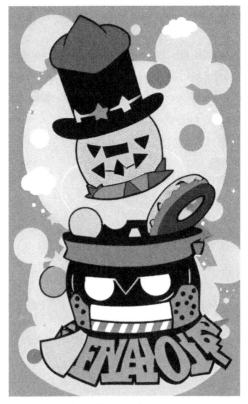

HAUNTED HEX

The Haunted Hex is a powerful and complex Voodoo spell that is designed to bring about intense feelings of fear and terror to the target. It is considered one of the most dangerous spells in Voodoo magic, as it has the potential to deeply affect the psyche of the target, causing long-term emotional trauma. The spell is typically used by practitioners seeking revenge or wishing to instill fear in their enemies.

The Haunted Hex is believed to have originated in New Orleans during the early 1800s. According to legend, a powerful Voodoo queen named Agassou created the spell to protect herself and her followers from those who sought to do them harm. The spell was said to be so potent that it could turn even the bravest of men into a quivering mass of fear.

However, the true power of the spell was not fully realized until many years later when it was used against a wealthy plantation owner who had mistreated his slaves. The slaves, desperate for revenge, turned to the Voodoo queen for help. In response, Agassou crafted the Haunted Hex and cast it upon the plantation owner.

The effects of the spell were immediate and devastating. The plantation owner was consumed by fear and terror, unable to sleep or eat for days on end. His mental state deteriorated rapidly until he was finally driven to madness. He was

eventually found dead, huddled in the corner of his bedroom, with a look of abject terror frozen on his face.

The story of the Haunted Hex quickly spread throughout New Orleans, and many began to fear the power of Voodoo magic.

You will need the following:

- A black candle
- A white candle
- A voodoo doll (representing the target)
- A piece of parchment paper
- A black pen
- A piece of the target's clothing or personal item
- Graveyard dirt
- A cauldron or fireproof bowl
- A black cloth
- A piece of hair from a black cat

To perform the spell, follow these steps:

1. Begin by lighting both the black and white candles and placing them in front of you.
2. Take the voodoo doll and place it on the parchment paper.
3. Using the black pen, write the name of the target on the parchment paper.
4. Take the piece of clothing or personal item from the target and place it on top of the voodoo doll.
5. Sprinkle some graveyard dirt on top of the voodoo doll and the clothing or personal item.
6. Light the piece of hair from the black cat and drop it into the cauldron or fireproof bowl.

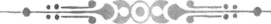

7. As the hair burns, recite the following incantation: "Spirits of the dead, hear my plea. Bring fear and terror upon my enemy. Let their soul be haunted day and night Until they are consumed by fright."

8. After reciting the incantation, place the parchment paper with the voodoo doll, clothing or personal item, and graveyard dirt into the cauldron or fireproof bowl.

9. As the parchment paper burns, focus your energy on the target, imagining them being consumed by fear and terror.

10. Once the parchment paper has burned completely, extinguish the black candle.

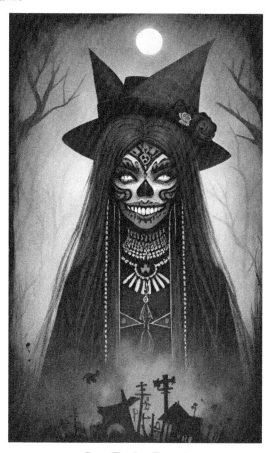

VENGEFUL VOODOO DOLL

The Vengeful Voodoo Doll is a powerful tool in the practice of voodoo magic, used to inflict harm or revenge upon an individual. It is believed that by creating a physical representation of a person, one can manipulate their spiritual essence and cause them pain or suffering.

Legend has it that the Vengeful Voodoo Doll originated from a powerful sorceress who sought to exact revenge on those who had wronged her. She believed that by creating a physical representation of her target, she could tap into their spiritual essence and cause them harm.

Over time, the practice of using voodoo dolls for revenge and justice became widespread, with practitioners using them to inflict physical pain or emotional suffering upon their enemies.

However, the power of the Vengeful Voodoo Doll was not without consequence. Those who used them for ill intent often found themselves plagued by misfortune and bad luck, as the spirits of voodoo were not to be trifled with.

You will need the following:

- Red fabric
- Needle and thread
- Black thread
- Scissors

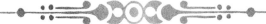

- Stuffing material (such as cotton or straw)
- Personal item or taglock from the target
- Black candle
- Salt
- Fireproof bowl

To perform the spell, follow these steps:

1. Begin by cutting a piece of red fabric into the shape of a human doll, approximately 6 inches in height.
2. Use the needle and thread to sew the edges of the fabric together, leaving a small opening at the bottom.
3. Turn the fabric right-side out, and stuff the doll with the chosen stuffing material.
4. Using the black thread, sew the opening at the bottom of the doll shut.
5. Take the personal item or taglock from the target, and attach it to the doll using the black thread.
6. Light the black candle and place it in the fireproof bowl.
7. Sprinkle a circle of salt around the candle.
8. Hold the doll over the candle and recite the following incantation:

   "By the power of the spirits of voodoo, I command this doll to carry out my will. Let the pain and suffering I feel be visited upon [target's name], and let them know the weight of their transgressions."

9. Visualize the target experiencing the suffering you wish to inflict upon them, and channel that energy into the doll.
10. Place the doll in a safe and secure location until the desired effect has been achieved.

CURSE OF THE SCORPION

The Curse of the Scorpion is a powerful hex in voodoo magic that is used to cause great harm to an individual. It is said that this curse is as potent as the sting of a scorpion, and can bring about great pain and suffering to the person it is cast upon.

Legend has it that the Curse of the Scorpion was originally created by a powerful voodoo priestess who sought revenge against her enemies. She captured a live scorpion and infused it with her powerful magic, creating a hex that was said to be as deadly as the venom of the scorpion itself.

Over the years, the curse has been passed down from generation to generation, and has become one of the most feared and respected hexes in voodoo magic. Its potency is said to be unmatched, and those who have been cursed with it are said to experience great pain and suffering until they either seek forgiveness or meet their ultimate demise.

You will need the following:

- A live scorpion
- Black candle
- Pinch of cayenne pepper
- Pinch of black pepper
- Pinch of salt
- Personal item belonging to the target (such as a strand of hair or piece of clothing)

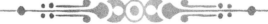

To perform the spell, follow these steps:

1. Begin by lighting the black candle and setting it on a flat surface.
2. Next, take the live scorpion and place it on the surface near the candle.
3. Sprinkle a pinch of cayenne pepper, black pepper, and salt over the scorpion.
4. Focus your intention on the person you wish to curse and recite the following incantation:

    "By the power of the scorpion's sting, Let this curse upon (target's name) bring. May pain and suffering be their fate, Until they beg for mercy at my gate."

5. Once you have recited the incantation, take the personal item belonging to the target and place it near the scorpion.
6. Watch as the scorpion crawls over the item, infusing it with the curse.
7. Once the scorpion has made contact with the personal item, pick it up and place it in a small container.
8. Keep the container in a dark, secluded area for seven days, allowing the curse to grow in strength.
9. After seven days have passed, release the scorpion into the wild, symbolically releasing the curse upon the target.

CURSED LEGACY

Cursed Legacy is a powerful voodoo spell that is designed to curse the legacy of a family or bloodline. This spell is believed to bring misfortune and chaos upon the descendants of the targeted family, causing their fortunes to wither away and their lives to be filled with suffering and despair.

The origins of the Cursed Legacy spell can be traced back to the early days of voodoo in Africa. Powerful shamans used the spell to curse rival tribes and their descendants in order to gain an advantage in territorial disputes and battles for resources.

Over time, the spell made its way to the New World, where voodoo practitioners adopted and modified it in Haiti and Louisiana. In these regions, the spell became a favorite of powerful voodoo queens and practitioners, who used it to curse their enemies and gain political power.

However, as the spell gained notoriety, some voodoo practitioners began to question its morality and its long-term effects. Many believed that the curse would eventually come back to haunt the caster, causing their own bloodline to suffer the same fate as their intended target.

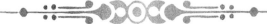

You will need the following:

- A black candle
- A piece of parchment paper
- A black pen
- A drop of the caster's blood
- Dirt from a cemetery
- A photo or personal item from the targeted family
- A cauldron or fireproof bowl
- A black cloth

To perform the spell, follow these steps:

1. Begin by lighting the black candle and placing it in the cauldron or fireproof bowl.
2. Write the name of the targeted family on the parchment paper using the black pen.
3. Place the photo or personal item from the targeted family on the parchment paper.
4. Add a drop of the caster's blood to the parchment paper.
5. Sprinkle some dirt from a cemetery on top of the parchment paper.
6. Fold the parchment paper three times and place it in the cauldron.
7. As the parchment paper burns, recite the following incantation:

   "By the power of the spirits of the dead, I curse the bloodline of [targeted family name]. May their lives be filled with pain and dread, And their legacy forever be stained."
8. Blow out the black candle and recite the incantation, then wrap it in the black cloth.

   "Black spirits and white, red spirits and gray, Mingle, mingle, mingle, you that mingle may! By the pricking of my thumb, Something wicked this way comes!"

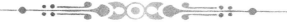

BONE SHAKER HEX

The Bone Shaker Hex is a powerful voodoo spell that is used to bring misfortune and chaos to an individual's life. It is a complex and dangerous spell that requires a deep understanding of voodoo magic.

The Bone Shaker Hex has a long history in voodoo magic. It is said that the spell was first created by a powerful voodoo priestess named Kalfa. She used the spell to bring down her enemies and protect her community from harm.

Over time, the spell evolved and became more powerful. It is now considered one of the most dangerous spells in voodoo magic. Some voodoo practitioners believe that the Bone Shaker Hex can only be cast by those with a deep understanding of voodoo magic, while others believe that anyone can use the spell with the right ingredients and incantation.

There is a story told among voodoo practitioners about a young woman who used the Bone Shaker Hex to get revenge on her cheating lover. She followed the spell exactly, burying the remains of the voodoo doll in a cemetery. But soon after, strange things began to happen. Her lover's life was turned upside down. He lost his job, his car, and his friends. Eventually, he became sick and died.

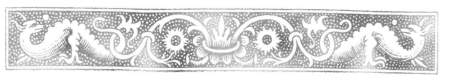

The young woman was haunted by guilt for the rest of her life. She realized too late that the Bone Shaker Hex was not something to be taken lightly. The spell had a life of its own, and once it was cast, it could not be undone.

You will need the following:
- A black candle
- A small voodoo doll made of straw or cloth
- A lock of hair or personal item from the target
- A piece of parchment paper
- A black pen
- Graveyard dirt
- A cauldron or fireproof bowl
- A black cloth

To perform the spell, follow these steps:

1. Begin by lighting the black candle and placing it in the cauldron or fireproof bowl.
2. Write the name of the target on the parchment paper using the black pen.
3. Place the lock of hair or personal item from the target on the voodoo doll.
4. Sprinkle some graveyard dirt on the voodoo doll.
5. Place the voodoo doll on the parchment paper.
6. Light the voodoo doll on fire, and place it in the cauldron or fireproof bowl.
7. As the voodoo doll burns, recite the following incantation: "Bone Shaker Hex, with this flame, Bring chaos to [target's name] name Shake their bones and rattle their soul. Make their life a living hell, take control."
8. Let the voodoo doll burn completely.
9. Wrap the ashes and remnants of the voodoo doll in the black cloth.
10. Bury the cloth in a cemetery or place it at a crossroad.

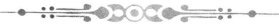

NECROTIC NUISANCE HEX

The Necrotic Nuisance hex is a powerful and malevolent voodoo spell used to inflict great harm and discomfort on the target. It is believed that this hex can cause the target to suffer from a range of physical and emotional ailments, including insomnia, chronic pain, and depression.

According to legend, a powerful voodoo queen created the hex to punish those who had wronged her or her followers. She would gather graveyard dirt, dried herbs, and powdered bones from the local cemetery and combine them in a cauldron with a lock of hair or personal item from the target. She would then light a black candle and recite the incantation, calling upon the spirits of the dead to inflict the target with a range of physical and emotional ailments.

Over time, the Necrotic Nuisance hex became one of the most feared spells in voodoo magic. It was said that those who fell under its curse would suffer from chronic pain, insomnia, and depression and that there was no known cure. Some even believed that the curse could be passed down through generations, affecting the target's descendants for years to come.

You will need the following:

- A black candle
- A piece of parchment paper
- A black pen

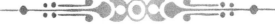

- A lock of hair or personal item from the target
- A mixture of graveyard dirt, dried herbs, and powdered bones
- A cauldron or fireproof bowl
- A black cloth

To perform the spell, follow these steps:

1. Begin by lighting the black candle and placing it in the cauldron or fireproof bowl.
2. Write the name of the target on the parchment paper using the black pen.
3. Place the lock of hair or personal item from the target on the parchment paper.
4. Sprinkle the mixture of graveyard dirt, dried herbs, and powdered bones on top of the parchment paper.
5. Fold the parchment paper three times and place it in the cauldron.
6. As the parchment paper burns, recite the following incantation:

   "Necrotic Nuisance, dark and vile, Inflict your curse on [target's name] with guile. Bring insomnia, chronic pain, and woe, Until [target's name] feels they cannot go."

7. Let the candle burn down completely, and then bury the remains of the spell in a graveyard or other sacred ground.

HELLFIRE HAZE HEX

The Hellfire Haze hex is a powerful curse that unleashes a cloud of toxic fumes that can cause extreme discomfort and pain to the victim. This hex is designed to make the target feel like they are in the depths of hell, surrounded by fire and brimstone.

It is said that the hex was created by a powerful voodoo queen who was betrayed by her lover. In revenge, she cast the hex on him, causing him to feel like he was burning alive. However, the hex went wrong, and the voodoo queen was also consumed by the Hellfire Haze. Her spirit still lingers in the toxic fumes, waiting for a new victim to curse. Be careful when casting this hex, as it is known to backfire and cause harm to the caster as well. Use it at your own risk.

You will need the following:

- Sulfur
- Chili peppers
- Garlic
- Snake venom
- Black candles
- A small pot

To perform the spell, follow these steps:

1. Start by lighting the black candles in a quiet and dark room. The candles should be arranged in a circle around the pot.
2. Place the sulfur, chili peppers, and garlic in the pot and light them on fire.

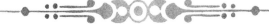

3. Add a few drops of snake venom to the mixture and let it simmer.
4. Close your eyes and focus on the person you want to curse. Chant the following incantation:

   "By the power of fire and venom, I curse you with the Hellfire Haze. May the toxic fumes of the underworld consume your body and soul. May you feel the burn of a thousand suns, and may your suffering be eternal."

5. Visualize the cloud of toxic fumes rising from the pot and surrounding the victim.
6. Blow out the candles and dispose of the pot far away from your home.

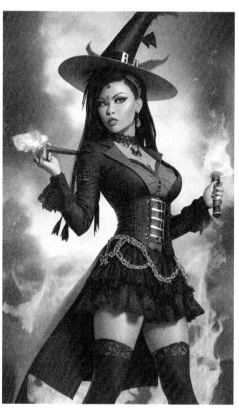

BANE OF THE BETRAYER

Bane of the Betrayer is a powerful Voodoo hex that is used to punish those who have betrayed you.

Legend has it that Bane of the Betrayer was first created by a powerful Voodoo priestess who had been betrayed by her lover. In her rage and desperation, she sought to create the ultimate punishment for those who dared to betray the trust of others. The hex was passed down through generations of Voodoo practitioners, and its power grew with each use.

However, the twist in the story is that the hex eventually turned on its creators. It is said that those who use the hex too often or for trivial reasons will be haunted by the spirits of the dead, who will seek revenge for the misuse of their power. Some even claim that the hex has a mind of its own and will turn on its user if they are not careful.

You will need the following:

- Black candles
- Dragon's Blood resin
- Graveyard dirt
- Black pepper
- Cayenne pepper
- Devil's Claw root
- Poppy seeds
- Mandrake root
- Snake skin

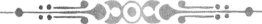

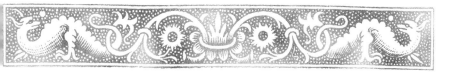

To perform the spell, follow these steps:

1. Light the black candles and focus on your intent to punish the betrayer.
2. Sprinkle the graveyard dirt around the candles.
3. Mix the Dragon's Blood resin, black pepper, cayenne pepper, Devil's Claw root, poppy seeds, and mandrake root together in a bowl.
4. Add snakeskin to the mixture and stir it clockwise while reciting the incantation: "By the power of the spirits of the dead, let the betrayer feel the pain of their misdeeds."
5. Take a small amount of the mixture and sprinkle it over the candles.
6. Light the mixture on fire and let it burn down completely, speaking the incantation.

   "By the power of Baron Samedi and the loa, I call upon the spirits of the dead to bring retribution upon the betrayer. Let them suffer the consequences of their actions and know the pain they have caused."

7. Collect the ashes and bury them in a graveyard, preferably on the betrayer's property.

REVENGE OF THE FORSAKEN

Revenge of the Forsaken is a powerful hex in Voodoo magic that is believed to bring justice to those who have been wronged. This spell is intended to exact revenge on an individual who has caused harm to the caster or someone they know.

The *Revenge of the Forsaken* hex has been used for centuries in Voodoo magic to bring justice to those who have been wronged. It is said to have originated in Haiti, where it was used by slaves to exact revenge on their cruel masters. Over time, the hex became more widespread, and it is now used by Voodoo practitioners all over the world.

The story tells of a young woman who was wronged by her lover. He had cheated on her with another woman, and the young woman was devastated. She turned to Voodoo magic for revenge and used the *Revenge of the Forsaken* hex to curse her lover. The hex worked, and her lover suffered greatly. However, as time passed, the young woman realized the error of her ways and regretted what she had done. She sought the help of a Voodoo priestess to reverse the hex, but it was too late. The damage had already been done, and the young woman was haunted by the guilt of her actions for the rest of her life.

It is a complex spell that requires great skill and knowledge of Voodoo magic.

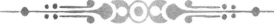

You will need the following:

- A black candle
- A poppet made of black cloth
- Black pepper
- Chili powder
- Ground cinnamon
- Ground cloves
- Garlic cloves
- An item belonging to the target (such as a piece of clothing or a lock of hair)
- Needle and thread
- Black ribbon

To perform the spell, follow these steps:

1. Light the black candle and place it in front of you.
2. Take the poppet made of black cloth and fill it with black pepper, chili powder, ground cinnamon, and ground cloves.
3. Add the garlic cloves and the item belonging to the target to the poppet.
4. Sew the poppet shut with the needle and thread.
5. Hold the poppet in your hand and recite the following incantation:
   "O spirits of the Voodoo faith, Hear my plea and bring me justice. Let the betrayer feel my wrath, And let them suffer for their unjustness."
6. Tie the black ribbon around the poppet and say:
7. "With this ribbon, I bind you tight. May you suffer day and night. Your punishment will be swift and sure, And justice will be served, pure and pure."
8. Bury the poppet in the ground or throw it into running water.
9. Blow out the black candle and say:
   "So hex it be."

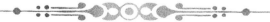

DIABOLICAL DEMISE HEX

This is a powerful voodoo spell that, if cast correctly, will bring pain and suffering to your enemies. Beware, though, as it is a spell not to be taken lightly, as it carries a heavy price.

It is said that it was created by a powerful voodoo queen in Haiti many years ago. She was known for her cruelty and her ability to inflict pain on her enemies using the most gruesome methods. The Diabolical Demise hex was her most feared spell, and she only used it in extreme cases, as it was believed to bring a curse upon whoever cast it.

Legend has it that one day, the voodoo queen decided to cast the hex on her own daughter, who had betrayed her. She followed the steps of the spell carefully, but as she chanted the incantation, something went terribly wrong. The spirits she had summoned turned against her, and the hex backfired, causing her to suffer an excruciating death.

You will need the following:

- A black candle
- Snake venom
- Powdered mandrake root
- Powdered sulfur
- An image of your enemy
- A piece of parchment paper
- A black feather
- A voodoo doll representing your enemy

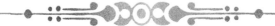

To perform the spell, follow these steps:

1. Light the black candle and place the image of your enemy next to it.
2. In a small bowl, mix a few drops of snake venom with powdered mandrake root and powdered sulfur until you have a thick paste.
3. Take the parchment paper and write the name of your enemy three times on it, then fold it three times.
4. Dip the black feather in the paste and use it to draw a pentagram on the folded parchment paper.
5. Place the voodoo doll on top of the pentagram, then spread the rest of the paste on it.
6. Light the parchment paper with the candle flame and let it burn completely, focusing all your anger and hatred toward your enemy.
7. As the parchment paper burns chant the following incantation three times:

   "From the darkness of the night, Bring forth the spirits of fright. With this hex, I do decree, My enemy shall suffer eternally."

8. Blow out the candle and dispose of the ashes and the voodoo doll.

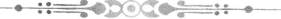

DAMNED DOMINION HEX

The Damned Dominion hex is a powerful voodoo spell that allows the caster to gain control over the will of another. This hex should not be taken lightly as it can have serious consequences and may lead to negative karma.

One famous story about the Damned Dominion hex tells of a woman who used the spell to gain control over her husband. She wanted him to be completely devoted to her, but the spell had unintended consequences. The more control she gained over him, the more he became obsessed with her, eventually leading to his descent into madness and his untimely death.

Another story tells of a voodoo priestess who used the Damned Dominion hex to control the local government officials. She was eventually discovered and imprisoned for her crimes, but the spell had already caused irreparable damage to the community.

You will need the following:

- A black candle
- Black pepper
- Graveyard dirt
- A piece of the target's hair or a personal item
- A black cloth
- A rusty nail

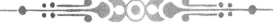

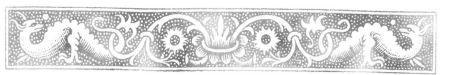

To perform the spell, follow these steps:

1. Light the black candle.
2. Sprinkle black pepper and graveyard dirt around the candle.
3. Take the personal item or hair of the target and place it in front of the candle.
4. Focus on the target and chant the following incantation: "Spirits of the dead, hear my plea, Give me power, give me thee. Bend the will of (target's name) to mine. Let them do as I design."
5. Take the rusty nail and pierce the personal item or hair of the target.
6. Wrap the personal item or hair in the black cloth and tie it tightly.
7. Let the candle burn out completely.

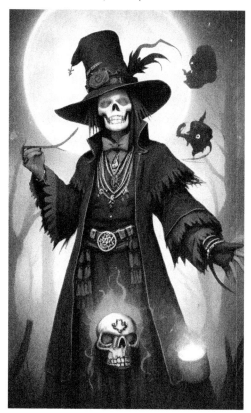

ETERNAL SUFFERING

This spell is not for the faint-hearted, as it is intended to inflict unimaginable pain and suffering on the victim for an indefinite period.

Legend has it that the spell was first created by a powerful Voodoo queen who sought revenge on her lover for betraying her. She performed the ritual with such ferocity that it inflicted eternal suffering on her lover and cursed her bloodline for generations to come. It is said that the curse still exists to this day and those who perform the spell risk the wrath of the Voodoo queen's spirit.

However, there is a twist to this tale. It is believed that the Voodoo queen herself fell victim to the spell she had created, as her lover was not the only one she had betrayed. She had also stolen a powerful talisman from a rival Voodoo priestess, who had vowed revenge. The priestess had secretly cast a spell on the talisman, which would activate if anyone tried to use it for their own gain. The Voodoo queen unknowingly used the talisman in the Eternal Suffering ritual, triggering the curse and dooming her to an eternity of suffering. Some say that her spirit still wanders the earth seeking revenge on those who dare to use her creation for their own purposes.

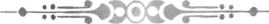

You will need the following:
- One black candle
- A pinch of graveyard dirt
- 13 black feathers
- The hair or fingernail clippings of the victim
- A piece of black fabric or cloth
- A small mirror
- A cauldron or large bowl
- A piece of paper and a pen
- Your own blood (optional)

To perform the spell, follow these steps:

1. Set up your altar by placing the black candle at the center, surrounded by the graveyard dirt and black feathers.
2. Place the victim's hair or fingernail clippings in the small mirror and cover it with the black cloth.
3. Light the candle and recite the following incantation three times: "Malfini, powerful spirit of the crossroads, I call upon you to lend me your strength and grant my wish. Bring eternal suffering to [victim's name], make them feel the pain they've caused me tenfold."
4. Take the mirror covered in black cloth and place it inside the cauldron or bowl.
5. Write the victim's name on the piece of paper and place it inside the cauldron as well.
6. If you're using your own blood, prick your finger with a needle or sharp object and drop a few drops into the cauldron.
7. Chant the incantation again while visualizing the victim writhing in pain and agony.
8. Blow out the candle and leave the cauldron on your altar for three nights. During this time, meditate on your intention and imagine the victim suffering.
9. After three nights, bury the contents of the cauldron in a graveyard.

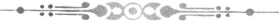

CURSED CROSSROADS

Cursed Crossroads is a powerful Voodoo magic hex used to bring misfortune and bad luck to an individual or a group of people. The hex is cast by creating a special crossroads and calling upon the spirits of the crossroads to carry out the curse.

Legend has it that the first practitioner of this hex was a powerful Voodoo priestess who was wronged by a wealthy landowner. The priestess, who had been skilled in the art of Voodoo magic, created a powerful hex that would bring misfortune and ruin to the landowner's family for generations.

Over time, the hex was passed down from generation to generation, and it became one of the most feared curses in all of Voodoo magic. It is said that those who have been targeted by the hex have experienced a series of unfortunate events, such as losing their job, experiencing financial ruin, or having their relationships fall apart.

This hex is not to be taken lightly, as it can have long-lasting and devastating effects on the target.

You will need the following:
- Black candles (4)
- White candles (4)
- Salt
- Black cloth
- A black chicken or rooster (alive)

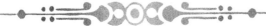

- A large knife
- Red pepper
- Garlic
- Black ink
- A piece of paper
- A pen or quill

To perform the spell, follow these steps:

1. Find a crossroads in a deserted area at night. It is essential that there are no cars or people around, as this may interfere with the hex.
2. Clear the area of any debris or trash, making sure it is completely clean.
3. Lay the black cloth on the ground to mark the crossroads. Use the salt to draw the outline of the crossroads on the cloth.
4. Place the black candles at the four corners of the crossroads and light them.
5. Use the knife to sacrifice the black chicken or rooster, sprinkling its blood around the crossroads.
6. Mix the red pepper, garlic, and black ink in a bowl, stirring it with the chicken's feathers. This mixture will be used to write the curse on the paper.
7. Write the name of the target on the paper with the pen or quill. Use the mixture from the bowl to write the curse, being sure to be as specific and detailed as possible.
8. Place the paper at the center of the crossroads and recite the following incantation:
   "Spirits of the crossroads, I call upon you. Bring misfortune and bad luck to (name of target). Let them feel the weight of your wrath and the power of this hex. So be it."
9. Blow out the candles and leave the crossroads, making sure not to look back.

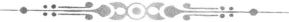

BITTER REVENGE BREW

Bitter Revenge Brew is a potent concoction used in Voodoo magic to exact revenge on one's enemies. This brew is not to be taken lightly, as it contains powerful magical ingredients that can cause harm if not used with caution.

One particular story tells of a man who angered a dark priestess by refusing to pay for her services. In retaliation, she created a batch of *Bitter Revenge Brew* and gave it to the man, telling him it was a gift. The man drank the brew and immediately fell ill, suffering from a mysterious illness that no doctor could cure. It wasn't until he returned to her and begged for her forgiveness that she lifted the curse and cured him.

The recipe for *Bitter Revenge Brew* has been passed down through generations of Voodoo practitioners and is considered one of the most powerful spells in their arsenal.

You will need the following:

- One black candle
- One bottle of dark rum
- 3 fresh limes
- One tablespoon of cayenne pepper
- One tablespoon of black pepper
- One tablespoon of dried thyme
- One tablespoon of ground ginger
- One tablespoon of dried rosemary
- One tablespoon of dried basil

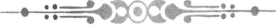

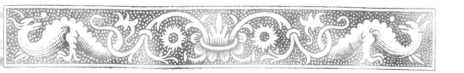

- One tablespoon of dried oregano
- One tablespoon of ground allspice
- One tablespoon of ground cinnamon
- One tablespoon of ground nutmeg
- One tablespoon of ground cloves
- One small piece of mandrake root
- One small piece of graveyard dirt

To perform the spell, follow these steps:

1. Begin by cleaning and purifying your workspace. Light a black candle and burn some sage to cleanse the area of negative energy.
2. Take the bottle of dark rum and pour it into a large cauldron or pot.
3. Squeeze the juice from the three fresh limes into the cauldron, stirring as you do so.
4. Add the cayenne pepper, black pepper, dried thyme, ground ginger, dried rosemary, dried basil, dried oregano, ground allspice, ground cinnamon, ground nutmeg, and ground cloves to the cauldron.
5. Stir the mixture clockwise nine times, chanting the incantation: "By the power of the spirits, let my enemies feel my wrath. Let this brew bring them misery and suffering."
6. Add the small piece of mandrake root and the small piece of graveyard dirt to the cauldron, stirring once more.
7. Let the mixture simmer over low heat for three hours, stirring occasionally.
8. Remove the cauldron from the heat and let the brew cool.
9. Once the brew has cooled, strain it through a cheesecloth or fine mesh strainer and pour it into a glass bottle or jar.
10. Seal the bottle or jar with a black candle wax and keep it in a cool, dark place until ready to use.

ACCURSED AFTERSHOCK

Accursed Aftershock is a powerful Voodoo spell that is used to curse an enemy with a devastating shock. The spell is designed to cause great harm and suffering to the target and is only used in extreme situations where all other options have failed. The curse is said to be so powerful that it can cause physical pain and even death, making it one of the most feared spells in the Voodoo tradition.

It is said to have originated in Africa, where tribes used it to curse their enemies and protect their land from invaders. Over time, the spell was brought to Haiti and other parts of the Caribbean, where it was refined and perfected by Voodoo priests and priestesses.

Legend has it that one particularly powerful Voodoo priestess used the Accursed Aftershock spell to defeat an entire army of enemy soldiers. She cursed them with the spell, and they were struck down by a terrible shock, causing them to flee in terror. From that day on, the spell became known as one of the most powerful curses in the Voodoo tradition.

However, it is said that the spell comes with a heavy price. Those who use it risk angering the spirits and inviting their wrath. Many Voodoo practitioners believe that the spirits will turn on those who use the spell, causing them to suffer a fate worse than death. As such, the spell is only used in the

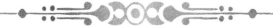

most extreme circumstances and only by those who are willing to risk everything.

You will need the following:

- A black candle
- A voodoo doll of the target
- A small piece of paper
- A pen or pencil
- Black pepper
- Salt
- A piece of black cloth
- A black string
- A lock of hair from the target

To perform the spell, follow these steps:

1. Begin by lighting the black candle and placing it in front of you.
2. Take the voodoo doll of the target and hold it in your hands. Visualize the target in your mind and focus on the anger and hatred that you feel towards them.
3. Take the piece of paper and write the target's name on it. Then, sprinkle black pepper and salt over the paper.
4. Fold the paper three times and then place it inside the voodoo doll. Visualize the curse taking hold of the target and causing them great pain and suffering.
5. Take the lock of hair from the target and tie it around the voodoo doll's neck with the black string. Make sure it is secure and tight.
6. Wrap the voodoo doll in the black cloth and tie it with the remaining black string. Make sure it is completely covered and secure.
7. Hold the wrapped voodoo doll in front of you and say the following incantation three times:

"By the power of the spirits and the force of the night, I call upon the ancient forces to curse my foe with all their might. May the shock of my curse be felt by the target like a bolt of lightning, May their pain and suffering be great, and may their spirit be forever frightening. Let this curse be a warning to all who dare to cross me, For the power of Voodoo will always set me free."

8. Once you have finished the incantation, extinguish the candle and bury the wrapped voodoo doll in a secret place where no one can find it.

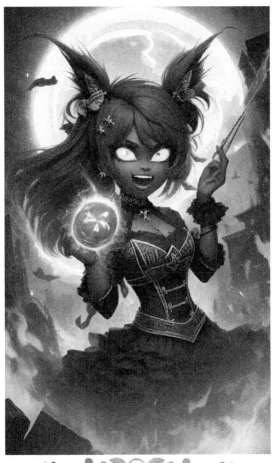

HEX OF THE HOWLING WIND

Hex of the Howling Wind is a powerful voodoo spell that harnesses the energy of the wind to bring about great change. This spell is particularly effective when used to bring justice or revenge upon one's enemies. The ritual requires careful preparation, and the spellcaster must be experienced in the art of voodoo magic.

You will need the following:

- A black candle
- A white candle
- A small amount of graveyard dirt
- A feather from a bird of prey
- A piece of black cloth
- A length of black string
- A small quantity of sulfur
- A small quantity of cayenne pepper
- A vial of dragon's blood oil

To perform the spell, follow these steps:

1. Begin the ritual on a windy night, preferably during a full moon. Set up your ritual space in a quiet, secluded area outdoors. Place the black candle to your left and the white candle to your right.
2. Take a pinch of graveyard dirt and sprinkle it around the base of each candle. Light both candles and focus on the flame, letting your mind become still and clear.
3. Hold the feather in your right hand and the piece of black cloth in your left. Visualize the wind blowing fiercely around you, filling you with its power.

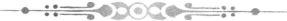

4. Begin to chant the following incantation slowly and deliberately:

   "Spirits of the wind, hear my plea. Carry my curse across land and sea. Let the power of the tempest guide This hex that I shall now provide."

5. Take the black cloth and wrap the feather inside it. Tie the black string around the bundle, knotting it three times. As you do this, visualize your enemy being bound and helpless, unable to escape the wrath of the wind.

6. Sprinkle sulfur and cayenne pepper over the bundle, sealing the curse within it. Dab a drop of dragon's blood oil on each knot to enhance the potency of the spell.

7. Hold the bundle up to the sky, letting the wind catch it and carry it away. As you watch it disappear into the night, say the following words:

   "By the power of the wind, this curse is cast. May the tempest wreak havoc, long and fast As I will, so mote it be."

8. Allow the candles to burn out completely. Bury the bundle of feathers, string, and cloth in a location where the wind is strong and unrelenting, far from your home.

SHADOWY SPECTER

Shadowy Specter is a powerful voodoo spell that calls upon a ghostly apparition to do your bidding. This spell requires a lot of focus, concentration, and some special ingredients. If you want to harness the power of the Shadowy Specter, be prepared to give up something of value to appease the spirits.

It is said that the spell was first used by a powerful voodoo queen who sought revenge against her enemies. The specter she summoned was so powerful that it haunted the entire village for generations, wreaking havoc on the descendants of those who wronged her.

However, the Shadowy Specter comes with a warning. It is a powerful spell that requires great sacrifice, and those who use it must be prepared to pay the price. Legend has it that the voodoo queen who first used the spell eventually became so consumed by the specter's power that she was unable to control it, and it ultimately consumed her.

You will need the following:

- A black candle
- A small mirror
- A lock of hair from the person you wish to haunt
- A personal item from the person you wish to haunt
- Graveyard dirt
- A piece of paper and a pen

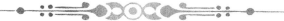

To perform the spell, follow these steps:

1. Begin by setting up your altar in a quiet, dimly lit room. Place the black candle at the center of the altar, and surround it with the mirror, lock of hair, personal item, and a handful of graveyard dirt.
2. Light the black candle and focus your energy on the flame. Visualize a shadowy figure emerging from the candle, taking form in the mirror.
3. Take the lock of hair and personal item, and hold them over the flame of the candle. As they burn, repeat the following incantation:

   "Shadowy specter, I call upon thee, To haunt this person eternally. With this sacrifice I make, Your power I humbly take. Rise from the darkness, heed my call, And do my bidding, one and all."

4. Take the piece of paper and write down your instructions for the shadowy specter. Be as specific as possible, outlining exactly what you want the specter to do.
5. Hold the paper over the candle flame and let it catch fire. As it burns, chant your instructions aloud, reinforcing your intention.
6. Blow out the candle, and let the smoke from the extinguished wick waft over the mirror. This will act as a conduit for the spirit to enter the physical realm.
7. Place the mirror in a safe place, away from prying eyes. Wait patiently for the specter to do your bidding.

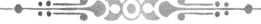

MALEVOLENT MIRAGE

Malevolent Mirage is a powerful Voodoo spell that creates a false reality around the target, causing them to experience a twisted, illusory world leading them further into despair. This spell can be used to punish those who have wronged you or to gain control over an individual by manipulating their perceptions of reality. However, it should be used with caution, as it has the potential to cause lasting psychological damage if misused.

Long ago, on the mystical island of Haiti, there lived a powerful voodoo priestess named Mambo Marie. She was revered by many in the community, as her spells had proven to be incredibly effective. Her most notable achievement was the creation of a powerful spell called Malevolent Mirage.

The spell was known for its ability to create a powerful illusion in the mind of its victim, making them believe that they were living out their worst fears. Mambo Marie kept the recipe for the spell a closely guarded secret for many years, only sharing it with her most trusted apprentices.

One day, a young apprentice named Jacques became enamored with the power that the Malevolent Mirage spell possessed. He begged Mambo Marie to teach him how to create the spell, promising that he would only use it for good. Against her better judgment, Mambo Marie eventually agreed to teach him.

But Jacques was not to be trusted. As soon as he had learned the spell, he began using it to manipulate and control those around him. People would do anything he asked out of fear that their worst nightmares would come true if they didn't comply.

Word of Jacques' powers quickly spread, and soon people began to fear him. He became known as the Malevolent Mirage Master, and many believed him to be invincible. But in reality, Jacques was consumed by his own fear and paranoia. He became increasingly isolated and paranoid, thinking that everyone was out to get him.

In a fit of desperation, Jacques used the Malevolent Mirag spell on himself, hoping to escape his fears. But the spell was too powerful, and he was trapped in his own personal hell for eternity.

You will need the following:

- Black candles
- Salt
- Black salt
- White sand
- Black tourmaline crystal
- Mandrake root
- White rose petals
- Mugwort
- Datura
- Belladonna

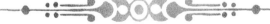

- Wormwood
- Hellebore
- Lemon balm
- Patchouli oil

To perform the spell, follow these steps:

1. Begin by creating a circle of salt around yourself and the target area.
2. Light the black candles around the perimeter of the circle and sprinkle black salt around the edges of the circle.
3. Place the black tourmaline crystal at the center of the circle and surround it with white sand.
4. Grind the mandrake root into a fine powder and sprinkle it over the sand and crystal.
5. Sprinkle white rose petals over the powder and add a pinch of mugwort, datura, belladonna, wormwood, and hellebore.
6. Light the patchouli oil and pass the smoke over the mixture, saying the incantation: "By the power of the spirits, let this mirage take form. Let it wrap around the mind of (target's name) and ensnare them in its hold."
7. Sprinkle lemon balm over the mixture and continue to chant the incantation until you feel the spell has taken hold.
8. Blow out the black candles and take down the circle of salt.

WRATHFUL WHIRLWIND

*W*rathful *W*hirlwind is a powerful voodoo spell that calls forth a destructive whirlwind to wreak havoc on your enemies. *J*t is said to have originated in the *W*est *A*frican country of *B*enin, where it was used by tribal leaders to protect their people from invading forces. *T*his spell is not for the faint of heart, as it requires a great deal of power and focus on performing successfully. *W*ith the right ingredients and incantations, however, you can harness the power of the wind to strike fear into the hearts of your foes.

You will need the following:

- A black candle
- A red candle
- A white candle
- A small mirror
- A black feather
- A white feather
- A small piece of paper
- Salt
- Black pepper
- Sandalwood incense
- A clear quartz crystal

To perform the spell, follow these steps:

1. Find a quiet, secluded area where you can perform the spell undisturbed.
2. Light the sandalwood incense and place it in a holder on the floor.
3. Place the black candle on the left side of the incense holder, the red candle on the right side, and the white candle in front of the incense holder.
4. Light the candles in the following order: white, black, and then red.
5. Take the black feather and wave it over the black candle, saying: "By the power of the wind, I call upon the spirits to heed my command."
6. Take the white feather and wave it over the white candle, saying: "By the power of the air, I command the winds to rise and obey me."
7. Take the small piece of paper and write the name of your enemy on it in black ink.
8. Sprinkle salt and black pepper on the paper, then fold it three times.
9. Hold the folded paper between your palms and say: "May the winds of the world carry my enemy away. May they be lost in the storm forevermore."
10. Place the folded paper on the small mirror and hold it up to the lit red candle, saying: "By the power of the elements, I command the winds to swirl and twist, to create a whirlwind of destruction that will engulf my enemy."
11. Hold the clear quartz crystal in your hand and focus your energy on it, visualizing the destructive whirlwind forming around your enemy.
12. Blow out the candles and the incense, then take the small mirror and bury it in the ground, preferably in a location where there is wind.
13. Leave the area and do not return for at least three days.

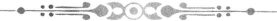

DEMONIC DOMINION

Demonic Dominion is a powerful and dangerous Voodoo spell granting the caster control over demons or other dark entities. This spell is not to be taken lightly and should only be used by experienced practitioners who fully understand the consequences of dabbling with the forces of the underworld.

You will need the following:

- Black candle
- Dragon's blood resin
- Myrrh resin
- Sandalwood incense
- Black salt
- Blood of a black rooster
- Small mirror
- Offering for the demon (optional)

To perform the spell, follow these steps:

1. Begin by creating a sacred space for your ritual. Cleanse the area with sage or other cleansing herbs and set up your altar. Place the black candle in the center of the altar and light it.
2. Sprinkle black salt around the candle in a circle, creating a protective barrier.
3. Light the sandalwood incense and let the smoke fill the room. This will help to purify the space and create a calm energy.
4. Take the mirror and place it in front of the candle. Make sure you can see your reflection in the mirror.
5. In a small dish, mix together the dragon's blood and myrrh resins. Light the mixture and allow the smoke to fill the room.

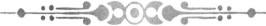

6. Take the blood of the black rooster and pour it into the dish with the smoking resins. Stir the mixture with a wooden spoon while reciting the incantation: "From the depths of darkness, I call forth thee, Demon of power and energy. By the blood of this rooster, I summon thee To do my bidding and fulfill my desire."

7. Take a few drops of the mixture and anoint the mirror with it. As you do this, repeat the incantation: "Mirror, mirror, on the wall. Show me the demon who will heed my call. Let me see him, let me know him, That I may command him."

8. Stare deeply into the mirror and visualize the demon coming forth from the underworld to do your bidding. Speak your desires clearly and with conviction, commanding the demon to do your will.

9. When you are finished, extinguish the candle and let the incense burn out. Thank the demon for its service (if you choose to offer an offering).

10. Dispose of the materials in a respectful manner, burying them in the ground or disposing of them in a body of water.

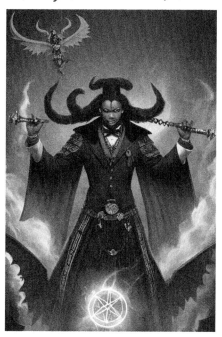

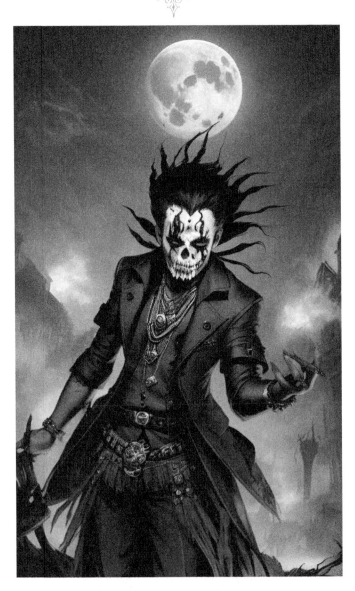

SINISTER SEANCE

Sinister Seance is a powerful Voodoo ritual that is used to communicate with the spirits of the dead. It is not a practice to be taken lightly, as it involves opening oneself up to the unknown and can be dangerous if not performed properly. This ritual has been used by Voodoo practitioners for centuries and is considered one of the most powerful forms of divination in the tradition.

The origins of Sinister Seance can be traced back to the early days of Voodoo in West Africa. It was believed that the spirits of the dead held great power and wisdom and that by communicating with them, one could gain insight into the future and guidance for the present.

You will need the following:

- A black candle
- A white candle
- A purple candle
- A small bowl of salt
- A small bowl of graveyard dirt
- A small bowl of powdered dragon's blood resin
- A small bowl of dried sage leaves
- A small bowl of dried mugwort leaves
- A small bowl of dried mandrake root
- A small bowl of dried wormwood leaves
- A small bowl of dried frankincense resin
- A small bowl of dried myrrh resin

- A small bowl of dried rose petals
- A small bowl of dried lavender flowers
- A small bowl of dried jasmine flowers
- A piece of an obsidian or black tourmaline crystal
- A piece of amethyst crystal

To perform the spell, follow these steps:

1. Begin by cleansing and purifying your workspace. Light the white candle and burn some sage to cleanse the area of negative energy.
2. Set up your altar with the black, white, and purple candles in a triangular formation. The black candle should be at the top point of the triangle, with the white and purple candles at the bottom corners.
3. Place the small bowl of salt at the base of the black candle, the small bowl of graveyard dirt at the base of the white candle, and the small bowl of powdered dragon's blood resin at the base of the purple candle.
4. Light all three candles, beginning with the black candle and moving clockwise around the triangle.
5. Sprinkle a pinch of each of the dried herbs and flowers onto the flames of each candle, one at a time, beginning with the black candle and moving clockwise around the triangle.
6. Place the obsidian or black tourmaline crystal at the base of the black candle and the amethyst crystal at the base of the purple candle.
7. Sit before the altar and close your eyes. Take several deep breaths, focusing on the candles and the energy they are producing.
8. When you are ready, chant the incantation: "Spirits of the dead, come to me. Hear my call and heed my plea. With this ritual, I summon thee. Show me what I seek to see."

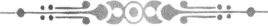

9. Visualize the spirits of the dead gathering around you, their energy mingling with yours. Keep your focus on the candles and the crystals as you continue to chant.
10. When you are ready to end the ritual, thank the spirits for their presence and extinguish the candles, beginning with the purple candle and moving counter-clockwise around the triangle.

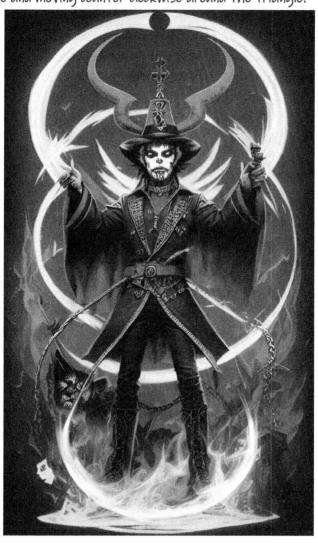

DEATH'S DOORWAY

*D*eath's *D*oorway is a powerful and dangerous *V*oodoo ritual that is used to communicate with the spirits of the dead and cross over to the other side. *T*his ritual is not for the faint of heart, as it involves making a direct connection with the spirit world and can be dangerous if not performed properly. *T*his ritual has been used by *V*oodoo practitioners for centuries and is considered one of the most powerful forms of divination in the tradition.

You will need the following:

- A black candle
- A white candle
- A red candle
- A small bowl of graveyard dirt
- A small bowl of powdered mandrake root
- A small bowl of dried mugwort leaves
- A small bowl of dried wormwood leaves
- A small bowl of dried frankincense resin
- A small bowl of dried myrrh resin
- A piece of an obsidian or black tourmaline crystal
- A piece of clear quartz crystal

To perform the spell, follow these steps:

1. Begin by cleansing and purifying your workspace. Light the white candle and burn some sage to cleanse the area of negative energy.
2. Set up your altar with the black, white, and red candles in a triangular formation. The black candle should be at the top point of the triangle, with the white and red candles at the bottom corners.
3. Place the small bowl of graveyard dirt at the base of the black candle, the small bowl of powdered mandrake root at the base of the white candle, and the small bowl of dried mugwort and wormwood leaves at the base of the red candle.
4. Light all three candles, beginning with the black candle and moving clockwise around the triangle.
5. Sprinkle a pinch of each of the dried herbs onto the flames of each candle, one at a time, beginning with the black candle and moving clockwise around the triangle.
6. Place the obsidian or black tourmaline crystal at the base of the black candle and the clear quartz crystal at the base of the red candle.
7. Sit before the altar and close your eyes. Take several deep breaths, focusing on the candles and the energy they are producing.
8. When you are ready, chant the incantation: "Death's Doorway, open wide. Hear my call, and be my guide. Take me to the other side, where the spirits and the dead reside."
9. Visualize the doorway to the spirit world opening before you, and the spirits of the dead beckoning you forward. Keep your focus on the candles and the crystals as you continue to chant.
10. When you are ready to end the ritual, thank the spirits for their presence and extinguish the candles, beginning with the red candle and moving counter-clockwise around the triangle.

GHOSTLY GRIEF

Ghostly Grief is a Voodoo ritual that is used to connect with the spirits of loved ones who have passed away. This ritual allows the practitioner to communicate with the spirit and express their grief, and can bring a sense of closure and peace to those who are mourning.

Ghostly Grief was a ritual that was commonly used by slaves and their descendants in the Americas to honor their ancestors and connect with the spirits of loved ones who had passed away. It was a way for them to maintain a connection to their African roots and continue to practice their ancestral traditions in a new land.

It is a powerful and emotional ritual that requires a deep connection to the spirit world.

You will need the following:

- A white candle
- A black candle
- A small bowl of graveyard dirt
- A small bowl of dried lavender
- A small bowl of dried rose petals
- A small bowl of dried chamomile
- A small bowl of dried yarrow
- A piece of clear quartz crystal
- A piece of rose quartz crystal
- A photo or object of the deceased

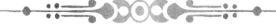

To perform the spell, follow these steps:

1. Begin by cleansing and purifying your workspace. Light the white candle and burn some sage to cleanse the area of negative energy.
2. Set up your altar with the white and black candles in a triangular formation. The white candle should be at the top point of the triangle, with the black candle at the bottom corner.
3. Place the small bowl of graveyard dirt at the base of the black candle and the small bowls of dried lavender, rose petals, chamomile, and yarrow at the base of the white candle.
4. Place the photo or object of the deceased in front of the white candle.
5. Light both candles, beginning with the white candle and moving clockwise around the triangle.
6. Sprinkle a pinch of each of the dried herbs onto the flames of the white candle, one at a time, beginning with the lavender and moving clockwise around the triangle.
7. Place the clear quartz crystal at the base of the white candle and the rose quartz crystal at the base of the black candle.
8. Sit before the altar and close your eyes. Take several deep breaths, focusing on the candles and the energy they are producing.
9. When you are ready, hold the photo or object of the deceased in your hands and chant the incantation: "Spirits of the dead, hear my call. Bring me comfort, ease my fall. Let me feel their presence near, And help me shed my earthly fear."
10. Visualize the spirit of the deceased appearing before you, and allow yourself to communicate with them. Express your grief and any other emotions you may be feeling. Allow yourself to feel their love and guidance.
11. When you are ready to end the ritual, thank the spirits for their presence and extinguish the candles, beginning with the black candle and moving counter-clockwise around the triangle.

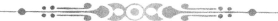

NECROMANCER'S NETWORK

Necromancer's Network is a powerful spell used in *Voodoo* magic to connect with the dead and communicate with them.

The *Necromancer's Network* spell dates back to ancient *Voodoo* traditions in *Africa*. *Powerful Voodoo* priests often used it to communicate with their ancestors and gain their wisdom and guidance. However, the spell became widely known in the 19th century when it was brought to the *United States* by *African* slaves. The spell was often used by slaves to communicate with their deceased loved ones and gain hope in their difficult lives.

One of the most famous stories surrounding the *Necromancer's Network* spell occurred in *New Orleans* in the early 20th century. A wealthy businessman who had lost his son to a tragic accident hired a *Voodoo* priestess to perform the spell in hopes of communicating with his son. The spell was successful, and the businessman was able to communicate with his son through the mirror. However, the businessman became obsessed with the spell and began to perform it every night, causing him to become weak and frail. Eventually, the businessman passed away, and it was rumored that his soul was trapped in the mirror, still communicating with his deceased son to this day. The mirror became known as the "*Necromancer's Mirror*" and was passed down through generations of *Voodoo* practitioners in *New Orleans*. It is

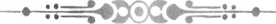

said that those who gaze into the mirror can still communicate with the businessman and his son, but at a great cost to their own souls.

This spell requires great caution and expertise as it is hazardous and can attract malevolent spirits if not performed correctly.

You will need the following:

- Black candle
- White chalk
- Anointing oil (preferably made from graveyard dirt, mugwort, and frankincense)
- A black obsidian crystal
- A white feather
- A small, sealed jar containing dirt from a cemetery
- A lock of hair from the person seeking to connect with the dead
- A small mirror

To perform the spell, follow these steps:

1. Start by marking a circle with white chalk on the ground. It should be large enough for you to sit inside.
2. Place the black candle at the center of the circle and light it.
3. Sit inside the circle and hold the obsidian crystal in your hand.
4. Use the anointing oil to draw a pentagram on the mirror.
5. Place the mirror in front of you and hold the lock of hair in your other hand.

6. Recite the following incantation: "Spirits of the dead, I call upon thee. Open the door between the living and the deceased. Hear my plea and grant me passage to the other side."
7. Blow out the candle and hold the mirror up to your face. Gaze into the mirror and focus on the lock of hair.
8. Say the name of the deceased three times while visualizing their face in the mirror.
9. Place the lock of hair and the white feather inside the jar of cemetery dirt.
10. Close the jar tightly and bury it in a cemetery.

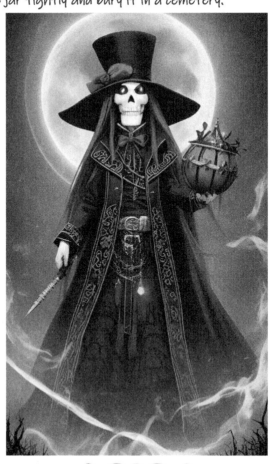

OUIJA ORACLE

Ouija Oracle is a powerful voodoo spell that allows you to communicate with the spirits of the dead.

The Ouija board has been used for centuries as a tool to communicate with the dead. Its origins can be traced back to ancient China, where it was used as a divination tool to communicate with spirits. The board as we know it today was first patented in the late 1800s and quickly became popular among spiritualists and occultists.

In voodoo, the Ouija board is used as a way to connect with ancestors and spirits of the dead. The board is seen as a powerful tool but also one that should be approached with caution. It is believed that if not used properly, the board can attract malevolent spirits that can cause harm to the user.

The Ouija Oracle spell is a powerful voodoo spell that should only be attempted by those with experience in working with spirits. It is not to be taken lightly, as it can open a portal to the spirit realm and attract entities that may not have your best interests at heart.

This spell is not for the faint of heart, as it involves the use of an Ouija board, which can be a conduit for both good and evil spirits.

You will need the following:

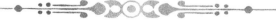

- Ouija board
- White candles
- Incense (frankincense, myrrh, or sandalwood)
- An object belonging to the deceased you wish to contact
- Salt
- Black cloth
- Protection talisman (e.g. black tourmaline)

To perform the spell, follow these steps:

1. Begin by setting up the Ouija board in a quiet, dimly lit room. Place white candles around the board and light them, along with the incense.
2. Sprinkle salt around the board in a clockwise direction to create a protective circle.
3. Sit at the board and place your hands lightly on the planchette.
4. Say the following incantation: "Spirits of the dead, I call upon thee. Come to me now and speak through me. Guide my hands and speak with clarity. Let us communicate in peace and harmony."
5. Focus your thoughts on the person you wish to contact and hold their object in your hands.
6. Ask your questions, allowing the spirits to guide the planchette to the letters and numbers on the board.
7. When finished, say, "Thank you, spirits. Go in peace and return to the realm of the dead."
8. Extinguish the candles and incense, and remove the salt from the room in a counterclockwise direction.
9. Wrap the Ouija board and object in a black cloth and keep it in a safe place until needed again.
10. Wear your protection talisman at all times to ward off any negative energies that may have been attracted during the communication.

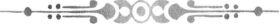

CEMETERY CONNECTION

Cemetery Connection is a powerful Voodoo spell that allows the caster to connect with the spirits of the dead who reside in a cemetery.

In the early days of voodoo, practitioners would visit graveyards and burial grounds in search of potent ingredients for their spells and communicate with the dead and gain insight into their lives and those around them. They would collect items such as graveyard dirt, bones, and other relics, which they believed held the power of the deceased.

Over time, the spell evolved to include personal items belonging to the deceased and the caster, as it was believed to strengthen the connection between the two worlds. However, it was also said that the spell could have unintended consequences if not performed correctly; inexperienced practitioners risked being possessed or harmed by malevolent entities. So practitioners were advised to use it with caution.

The spell requires a solid connection to the spirit world and an understanding of the spirits that inhabit the cemetery.

You will need the following:

- A black candle
- A piece of black cloth
- A small shovel

- Graveyard dirt
- A personal item belonging to the deceased
- A personal item belonging to the caster
- A piece of parchment paper
- A pen or quill
- A black ribbon

To perform the spell, follow these steps:

1. Find a quiet and secluded spot within the cemetery that resonates with you. Set up the black cloth and light the black candle in the center of it.
2. Using the small shovel, collect a small amount of graveyard dirt from around the base of a tombstone. Sprinkle it around the candle.
3. Place the personal item belonging to the deceased on the cloth next to the candle and the personal item belonging to the caster on the opposite side.
4. Take the piece of parchment paper and write the name of the deceased on it. Use the pen or quill to write your question on the paper as well.
5. Roll up the parchment paper and tie it with the black ribbon.
6. Hold the parchment paper in front of the candle and recite the following incantation three times: "By the power of the spirits that dwell in this place, I call forth the one who's left us without a trace. Guide me with your knowledge and lend me your sight. Answer my questions and bring your insight."
7. Place the parchment paper on the cloth in front of the candle and wait for a response from the spirits.
8. Once you receive an answer, thank the spirits for their guidance and blow out the candle.
9. Leave the personal item belonging to the deceased on the tombstone as a token of respect.

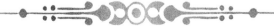

Printed in Great Britain
by Amazon

41068444R00086